MEDICAL AUDIT
AND
GENERAL PRACTICE

MEDICAL AUDIT
AND
GENERAL PRACTICE

Second Edition

Edited by

MARSHALL MARINKER

*Director of Medical Eduction, MSD, and
Visiting Professor of General Practice,
United Medical and Dental Schools of
Guy's and St Thomas's Hospitals*

BMJ
Publishing
Group

First published in 1995
by the BMJ Publishing Group, BMA House, Tavistock Square,
London WC1H 9JR

British Library Cataloguing in Publication Data

A catalogue record for this book is available
from the British Library

ISBN 0-7279-0908-8

Typeset, printed and bound in Great Britain by
Latimer Trend & Company Ltd, Plymouth

Contents

Advisory Editorial Board

Acknowledgments

It is a pleasure to express my thanks to so many friends and collaborators who have helped in the production of this second edition. Once again Dr Ian Bogle, Sir Michael Drury, and Dr Bill Styles joined me on the Editorial Advisory Team, and I owe much to their general wisdom and detailed and practical help. Also I wish to thank all the authors for their patience and forbearance in the rather long editorial process.

The Department of Health was generous in making a financial grant to the MSD Foundation towards the production of the first edition of this book, and true to its word in giving the editor free rein. MSD Ltd have been similarly generous in supporting this second edition, and equally scrupulous about editorial freedom.

Finally I should like to record my sincere thanks to Ms Deborah Reece, BMJ Books Editor, Ms Jane Sugarman, freelance copy-editor, and my secretary Ms Carolyn Lee.

MARSHALL MARINKER

Preface to second edition

This second edition has seen the updating of much of the original material, and the addition of new chapters which reflect the application of audit in a variety of recently created organisations and situations. Examples include the views from practice management, fundholders, and the FHSAs. In introducing this second edition, I want to take the opportunity to deal with two issues of what, in the current jargon, would be termed political correctness. The first refers to the meaning of "medical audit," the second to the link between medical audit and contracts.

In recent years a number of writers have sought to differentiate medical audit from clinical audit: medical audit is taken to be concerned exclusively with the behaviour of doctors, and clinical audit with the work of all those colleagues (including doctors) involved in the delivery of health care.

I take the view that this distinction is unhelpful, because in contemporary health care it is virtually impossible to envisage any aspects of quality that rely entirely on the performance of doctors, divorced from the collaboration, support, and often leadership of other colleagues. In this sense, the term "medical audit" in this book should be read as a synonym of "clinical audit."

The chapters of the first edition of this book were all written around the time of the publication of the Government's radical restructuring of the National Health Service. In 1990 we had only just been introduced to the separation of the purchasing and providing functions; to the setting up of trusts and fundholding practices; to a new contract for general practitioners which demanded detailed accountability for tasks and targets. All of this has created a large managerial appetite for what, in my opening chapter, I termed the contractual purposes of medical audit.

As purchasing authorities, fundholders, hospital trusts, and general practices strive to achieve cost benefit in the NHS, a growth industry has developed in defining packages of care, drug formularies, clinical guidelines, and patient charters. There is an attempt to measure the performance of the practice against public and published expectations, albeit expectations that seek to reflect the best evidence of good practice from current research. These demands of managed health care subtly colour and shade the characteristics of medical audit, so that it is in danger of becoming identified with external accountability.

If medical audit focuses on, or is restricted by, these managerial demands for accountability, something very important and precious will be lost from both medical audit and general practice. Of course public accountability is both managerially essential and morally desirable. But medical audit should first be seen as integral to the professionalism of all those who undertake health care. It is a tool for achieving for the practice what Schön urged on the practitioner—that reflection in action which is the surest guiding principle of good quality care.[1]

MARSHALL MARINKER
March 1995

1 Schön DA. *The reflective practitioner.* New York: Basic Books, 1983.

Preface to first edition

Medical audit is a promising means to an essential end—improving the quality of medical care that the patient receives. A commitment to medical audit has now been expressed by the major professional bodies concerned with clinical medicine in the National Health Service. None the less, anxieties remain. Will medical audit be simply a device for controlling the contract between the doctor and the state? What will be audited? Who will determine this? Who will write the standards? To whom are the auditors accountable? What will be the consequences for the professionalism of doctors, for the independence of the practice, for the standards of care that the patient will receive?

This book is designed for general practitioners who wish to embark on medical audit. It is concerned not only with the mechanisms of audit in general practice but also with its philosophy and intentions. Most of the authors are principals in general practice. They have described an approach to medical audit that is rooted in the experience of general practice. However stringently the present or future contracts of general practitioners are monitored by the health care authorities, appropriate standards of care must be identified, composed, and monitored effectively by those with direct responsibility for the care of patients.

Rudolph Klein,[1] commenting on the larger transformations of British society, wrote that in the 1980s the relationship between the professions and the public shifted from one based on status and trust to one based on contract. Nevertheless, in the past the achievements and success of British general practice have resulted not from the wording of contracts or the imposition of control but from the free exercise of professional good conscience. This book seeks to build on this professional good conscience by explaining the role of medical audit in the future development of each practice and of general practice as a professional discipline.

The intention has been to provide practical guidelines without being prescriptive: to leave room for the diversity, creativity, and energy which have ensured the best of practice and which, with the help of medical audit, can achieve so much more.

MARSHALL MARINKER
July 1990

1 Klein R. From status to contract: the transformation of the British medical profession. In: *Proceedings of Anglo-American Symposium on health care provision under financial constraint: a decade of change.* University of North Carolina, 1990.

Contributors

Graham Buckley, Director, Scottish Council for Postgraduate Medical and Dental Education

Sir Michael Drury, Emeritus Professor of General Practice, University of Birmingham

Brian M Goss, GP Fundholder, Bungay, Suffolk

Rosey Foster, Chief Executive, Association of Managers in General Practice, London

Sandra Gower, Practice Development Manager, Chairman, Association of Managers in General Practice, London

Jacqueline V Jolleys, Honorary Lecturer, Department of General Practice, University of Nottingham

Marshall Marinker, Director of Medical Education, MSD Ltd; Visiting Professor of General Practice, UMDS, London

Mike Pringle, Professor of General Practice, Department of General Practice, University of Nottingham

Kay Richmond, Principal Medical Officer, Health Professional Group, the Welsh Office, Cardiff

Daphne Russell, Director of Statistical Support Unit, University of Hull

Ian Russell, Founding Professor of Health Sciences, University of York

Brenda Sawyer, Practice Manager, Education Director, Association of Managers in General Practice, London; Research Fellow, Institute of General Practice, University of Exeter

Jonathan Shapiro, Senior Fellow, Health Services Management Centre, University of Birmingham

Bill Styles, Chairman of Council, RCGP; General Practitioner, London

Colin Waine, Director of Primary Care, Sunderland Health Commission

1 Principles

MARSHALL MARINKER

Creativity and error

Medical science, in common with all other sciences, depends on a balance, a congruity, and a collaboration between creativity and critique. If clinical medicine is to be scientific in its orientation and honesty general practitioners must be creative in their search for good standards of practice and their own sternest critics in searching for error.

The habit of truth is central to scientific endeavour. Perhaps the most powerful tool of modern science has been the pursuit of the null hypothesis. Here the task of scientists is to submit what they believe to be the truth to the most searching attack that evidence and logic can mount. They attempt to prove that what they have found is simply a chance event or random relationship, which has no general relevance or validity. The search for error is the crucial expression of the habit of truth. Yet much in medical education and medical practice teaches us to associate error with blame, and blame with shame and punishment. No wonder that we have little appetite to search for error.

It is possible to be active or passive in our efforts to suppress the truth or to fail to recognise it. I can hide the fact that I have prescribed a harmful medication, or failed to understand or act appropriately on the evidence to hand. That is active deceit. Of course my professional conscience will prick me. I may also fear the shame of discovery more than I fear the pain of confessing my fault. But at least my deceit is conscious and amenable to challenge.

But I can also fail to recognise error simply by refusing to search for it, by being over zealous in my compliance with current belief.

1

Much of my own education at medical school encouraged this professional good conduct. This is passive deceit, and it is much more dangerous than active deceit. It stunts the growth of knowledge; it strengthens authority and it paralyses creativity. And it does all this silently, because the professional conscience is anaesthetised by habit and conformity.

McKintyre and Popper[1] called for a new ethics of medical practice in which error would be valued, cherished even, as a major source of learning. They write:

> In monitoring medical care tolerance is essential and in the search for mistakes there should be no denigration of others nor any condemnation associated with the process of peer review. It would be morally wrong and would deter doctors from taking part. The goal must be educational and practical: it must be linked to the improvement of all doctors and not to the punishment of those who err. Only with such an ethos can we establish a new type of confidence: that mutual criticism is not personal and pejorative but that it springs from a mutual respect and a desire to improve the lot of patients.

As therapies become more powerful the public protects itself with more ambitious and punishing litigation. Those who hold the budgets for medical care (whether a government department or a private insurance company) demand tighter and tighter contractual controls over the performance of doctors. In this sense "error" and "deviations from contractual norms" may be dangerously confused. Medical audit is a means of searching for error. If it becomes only a tool for monitoring deviations from contractual norms it will have little to do with science and quality. McKintyre and Popper look foward to a robust independent profession so open to self critical analysis that the public will have little need for litigation, and the government will have less cause to impose tight contracts.

The search for error is part of the search for continuous improvement in health care. Berwick[2] examines the theory of quality improvement in industry and applies this to the practice of medicine. He writes:

> ... a test result lost, a specialist who cannot be reached, a missing requisition, a misinterpreted order, duplicate paperwork, a vanished record, a long wait for the CT scan, an unreliable on-call system—these are all-too-familiar examples of waste, rework, complexity, and error in the doctor's daily life. ... For the average doctor, quality fails when systems fail.

Berwick contrasts two approaches to the search for error. He calls the first the "theory of bad apples:" here the approach is punitive, and there are overtones of "recertification" or "deterrents" or "litigation." Of this approach he writes: "In fact, practically no system of measurement—at least none that measures people's performance— is robust enough to survive the fear of those who are measured."

The second approach that he describes is widely used in Japanese industry. It is called *kaizen*. In medical care *kaizen* would mean that every health care worker involved in a particular system would be encouraged and educated to improve performance. In place of punishment there would be a sense of discovery, pride, and achievement brought about by creative leadership. That is what we see in the best of British general practice today, and this book is written in the hope and expectation of encouraging just such an approach.

Coming to terms

In the literature of medical audit each author creates his own definition of the term, and each definition varies subtly from all those which went before. Let me then propose my own. *Medical audit is the attempt to improve the quality of medical care by measuring the performance of those providing that care by considering the performance in relation to desired standards, and by improving on this performance.* The reader will be immediately aware that every term used in my definition gives rise to further questions, rather than explanations. The opening two chapters of this book are concerned with the exploration of some of the questions raised and with a search for some further explanations.

The term "medical audit" has been with us for three decades. During that time it hs given rise to a burgeoning literature. A search through this literature reveals a number of other terms, used either as synonyms or to identify closely allied concepts. Terms such as "standard setting," "performance review," "peer review," and "quality assurance" have been coined to explain medical audit, to soften or sharpen the image, or to apologise for it.

An exponential growth of papers and books on any subject is more often a sign of hope, enthusiasm, and uncertainty than of success, benefit, and proof. Further, the enthusiasm for medical audit shown not only by clinicians and medical academics but also by politicians and Treasury civil servants may suggest that, although all the proponents may know what they are talking about, they are not necessarily talking about the same thing. Indeed, as this book will reveal, the implementation of medical audit embraces philosophical speculation and examination of moral values, a reinterpretation both of clinical teaching and of the logic of clinical problem solving, the numerical skills of epidemiology, the narrative skills of case discussion, and the political skills of negotiating change. All of these, at one time or another, must be employed in the course of medical audit.

As there are no universally accepted crisp and clear definitions of the terms used, no single purpose for the use of audit, no copper bottomed guarantees (backed by hard evidence) that the game is worth the candle, what then is the rationale for this book? Clearly the authors believe strongly in the value of medical audit. This belief alone, however, would scarcely constitute a defence for writing the book. That defence must rest on other supports—from logic, from experience, and from the results of research. Medical audit should be characterised by the discipline that it serves, by medicine itself. Medicine is more than a biotechnology. It is both art and science, philosophy and politics. The American sociologist Ashley Montague[3] wrote that medicine was neither an art nor a science in itself but rather a special sort of relationship between two people: the doctor and the patient. Unless medical audit impinges materially and beneficially on the clinical and social purpose of this relationship there will be little motivation to learn about it, to develop it, and to practise it.

Medical audit is not an end in itself. It is a tool to achieve a desired end. In fact medical audit refers to a number of tools, fashioned to achieve a number of different ends. These ends may be described as contractual, managerial, or educational. Inevitably there is an overlap of all three. Compliance with a contract is in fact a managerial imperative. All medical audit, no matter what its intentions, reveals something new to the auditor and so has educational value. Nevertheless, it may be useful to consider the differences between the contractual intentions of medical audit and the more imaginative use of audit as a guide to better clinical practice and practice management.

Contractual intentions

Audit for the purposes of contract is centrally concerned with compliance and control. The Family Health Services Authority (in

4

Scotland, Health Board) may seek to monitor a contract that specifies a range and levels of performance. Here medical audit may be used simply to provide evidence that the contract has been fulfilled, that the range and levels of performance have been attained, and therefore that appropriate payment can be made. In this form of audit no questions are raised about appropriateness, the benefit or cost of the audit, or the impact on the health of patients. The problems of medical audit for the purposes of contract might therefore appear to be simply mechanical. This appearance is misleading because in fact there are moral as well as technical problems to be tackled.

One important example, from the new National Health Service contract for general practitioners, will suffice. Cervical cytology is an invasive procedure. In the course of clinical problem solving there is an evident ethical duty on the part of the doctor to negotiate such invasive procedures. When such an invasive procedure is carried out not on a patient with a relevant medical problem but on a well person in the search for hidden disease this duty is made sharper and more urgent. Such negotiation would be difficult enough, even if the benefits from such screening could be securely demonstrated from scientific research. In fact, there is room for discussion and doubt.[4] The clinical significance of abnormal histology, apart from the finding of actual malignant change, remains uncertain. These so called abnormal findings may occur in up to 30% of specimens examined. There is no consensus about how to interpret them, or about what action should follow. There remain questions about cost/benefit—cost expressed not only in financial terms but in terms of the patient's anxiety and distress. To complete the list of dilemmas, the new contract rewards the general practitioner financially for obtaining high levels of compliance with the procedure, in a population of otherwise well persons.

The major difference between carrying out medical audit for the purposes of contract and carrying out audit to improve clinical care and practice management may be psychological. Contractual audit may appear to be regulatory and punitive rather than developmental. Nevertheless, it may serve as an introduction to "the real thing." As the mechanics of selecting, handling, and interpreting the data are similar, no matter what the purposes of the auditor, these contractual audits may be regarded as simple five finger exercises: a necessary rehearsal. There is a further benefit

5

to be gained from success in carrying out such contractual audits. Practice income can thus be maximised. Maximising practice income creates greater freedom and funds to improve the service to patients.

Audit for clinical and practice management

Medical audit is concerned with much more than fulfilling the terms of any current contract. It is concerned with the following issues: the range of services offered to patients; how and why these may change over time; what choices should be made about the use of limited resources; what standards of care should be aimed for and on what basis these standards will be created, judged, and revised. The role of control and compliance, so important in contractual audit, is secondary and subservient to these much more important priorities. The following tasks are required in an overall management audit strategy:

- Determining which aspects of current work are to be considered
- Describing and measuring present performance and trends
- Developing explicit standards
- Deciding what needs to be changed
- Negotiating change
- Mobilising resources for change
- Reviewing and renewing the process.

It will be clear that these seven tasks require an imaginative and creative approach to what it is that the practice is there to do. The development of general practice now demands, as never before, that partners and other members of the practice are given an opportunity to explore their ideas for the future, and to discover a strong sense of ownership of these ideas and enterprises. All the partners in a practice, and all the colleagues who work with them in the primary health care team, will be involved in one aspect or another of medical audit. All these tasks require sensitive and rigorous group work, and this is discussed further.

The practice of medical audit, like the practice of clinical science, demands a mixture of creativity and critical analysis. The auditors must therefore consider, in relation to anything that they are planning to do, what resources are needed. What *information* will be necessary to monitor events? A sound principle in determining what data are required is the principle of economy of effort. All too often enthusiastic auditors set about collecting and collating almost all the data available on their chosen topic. Later there is a discussion on the sampling of data and other ways of reducing the number of facts that must be looked for and processed. Consideration of the information required leads to choice of the *necessary technology*. The computer is becoming an indispensable tool of practice management and medical audit. Consideration must then be given to *personnel*: the various tasks of medical audit must be distributed among members of the practice in accordance with their aptitudes, their interests, and their commitment. Clear definition of tasks and responsibilities is essential, although these cannot be ascribed by dictate but must be negotiated. *Time* may be perceived by members of the practice as the most scarce resource. A realistic estimate of the time involved in medical audit is essential. Much has been written about the management of time, but time has to be "created" rather than "found." Creating time for medical audit involves a reallocation of some tasks, and perhaps the abandoning of others that have been kept going, not because they are particularly beneficial but because they are part of the practice's traditional way of working. Finally *space* must be found and allocated, and those responsible for the practice's budget must take account of the *financial cost*.

What can be measured or described?

Avedis Donabedian,[5] perhaps the most influential theorist in the field of quality assurance in health care, differentiates between three aspects of a health service: structure, process, and outcome.

Structure

Structure refers to the physical and personnel resources of an organisation. Examples would include the building, the number of rooms, and their size and use; the equipment that the practice employs; the number of patients and ratio of patients to doctors; the number and categories of other staff. Structure is perhaps the easiest to measure of the three components of health care. One of the first formal approaches to medical audit in general practice, that initiated by the Joint Committee on Postgraduate Medical Training,[6] relied heavily on such measurements. The relative ease with which structure can be measured is balanced by the relative difficulty—I would rather say near impossibility—of making other

7

than value judgments about them. These value judgments, however, are both inescapable and appropriate.

Process

Process refers to the actions taken by all those involved in the aspect of care that is being audited. Processes would include measurements of consultation rates, the items recorded in the records, the frequency of use of particular instruments, investigations carried out or referral to other health care personnel, the number and type of drugs prescribed, and the frequency and scale of the use of all other health care resources. It will be clear that the number of processes that can be measured in relation to any particular aspect of medical care is considerable, and choices must be limited by the resources available for measurement and interpretation. The measurement of process is the most common activity in medical audit. Medical audit as defined in the general practitioners' new contract is almost exclusively concerned with the measurement of process. Most of the audits described in this book rest largely on the measurement and interpretation of items of process.

Outcome

Outcome refers to the results of health care, and health care may be described as the product of the structures (the resources that are available) plus the processes (the activities of the health care workers concerned). These outcomes are expressed in terms of the patient's health status or physical or social function. Suicide and parasuicide rates might be used as an outcome measure of the success or failure of diagnosing and treating depression. School absence might be a useful outcome measure in assessing the diagnosis and management of childhood asthma.

Making judgments

Purists have argued that only an audit of outcome is worth while and that measures of structure and process are of value only if they can be shown to have a direct link with the outcome. Without the evidence of such a direct link, it is argued, it is impossible to know how either structures or processes should be changed. This purist view is certainly not supported by Donabedian, nor, I think, is it supported by logical analysis of the purposes and possibilities of medical audit.

As far as measurements of structure are concerned, value judgments may be made without too much embarrassment. Is it really necessary to demonstrate that a cold and cramped consulting room with poor sound insulation results in failures of diagnosis or deteriorations in health? The absence of an effective steriliser, a paucity of support staff, the lack of reference books in the consulting room, or of a practice library, may all be safely judged as having a negative influence on the quality of care.

Value judgments about process data rely in part on logic and common sense and in part on the results of previous good research. Both these reference points (common sense and research) although indispensable must be treated with some reserve. The common sense of one decade may appear nothing more than a passing fashion in the next. Most good research provides not only answers to clinical problems but fresh questions, a stimulus to new research, and the possibility that the previous answers will be found inadequate.

The judgments that flow from research can sometimes appear less securely anchored in hard evidence than judgments based on common sense and professional values. Twenty years ago research suggested that in children under the age of 3 years *Haemophilus influenzae* was a common cause of otitis media and therefore that phenoxymethylpenicillin (penicillin V) would be ineffective and a broader spectrum antibiotic should be employed. Since then much research has suggested that the use of antibiotics has little effect on the natural history of otitis media in children. A subsequent review article[7] suggests that perhaps after all there is a place for antibiotic therapy in the management of this condition.

Items of process such as the recording of risk factors—for example, drug idiosyncracies—in the patient's notes must self evidently appear to be a good thing. Their general absence from the practice's record system may be regarded with justified anxiety. Howie[8] chose to regard the prescribing of an antibiotic for children with upper respiratory tract infection as an indicator of poor care. His judgment was based on the results of a great deal of research, including his own, which suggests that such antibiotic treatment is relatively ineffective. In his paper Howie makes it clear that he is making a value judgment based in part on findings from research and in part on logic and extrapolation. This honesty allows others to come to a decision about how much credence they can give to his conclusions.

Another example of the use of process measures as an indicator of the quality of care concerns the routine monitoring of blood pressure measurement in the audit population, in the search for moderate to severe hypertension, long advocated[9] as one of the benchmarks of good preventive medicine in modern general practice. This judgment is based on much research that correlated hypertension with the incidence of stroke and established the benefits of controlling this hypertension.

The rub is that although measures of outcome are intellectually satisfying they are also quite rare. There are a number of reasons for this. So many factors affect the natural history of most medical conditions that it can be difficult to say that the outcomes observed were actually brought about, or materially affected, by the structures and processes desired. In spite of massive research into the surgery, radiotherapy, and chemotherapy of breast cancer, we still remain uncertain about the treatment of choice. To take another example, our knowledge of the causes, course, and management of lower back pain is so insubstantial that few would be prepared to make a firm link between the choice of therapy and the ensuing duration and severity of the symptoms.

Where good research has been able to establish firm links between process and outcome, measures of process can be accepted with some confidence as indicators of quality. An example would be evidence from glycosylated haemoglobin measurements that blood sugar is being well controlled in diabetics. We know from research that end organ damage is reduced when blood sugar is well controlled by diet and medication. Glycosylated haemoglobin measurements correlate strongly with levels of blood glucose control over long periods of time.

Populations and samples

For the most part medical audit refers to the monitoring of populations. It is a golden rule of medical audit, as of all empirical research, that the greatest benefit, in terms of what is to be learned, should be purchased for the smallest cost, in terms of the number of resources used and data collected. There may therefore be situations in which it would be both economical and morally acceptable to create a small representative sample from the total

10

number; for example, the practice might wish to check that the records of addresses and telephone numbers of its elderly patients are valid. Here sampling may be sufficient to provide evidence of overall practice performance in this area of documentation. The relationship between the size of the sample and the confidence we can have in the results of our findings, and the ways in which valid samples may be chosen, are considered by Ian and Daphne Russell in chapter 11.

When medical audit is used to improve the care of certain categories of patients the sample should contain all those patients known to have the same condition. The reasons for this are self evident. As we know from previous large population studies something about the prevalence of each condition in relation to the age/sex distribution of the practice population, the finding of a lower proportion of hypertensive, diabetic, or asthmatic individuals than might have been expected would provoke the questions: "How can we improve our early diagnosis of this condition?" "How can we improve the efficiency of our disease register?" In this kind of audit it is important to include in the population being studied all those patients who have the condition that is being audited. The reason is a practical one: if error is detected this can be rectified for the individual patient, whose care is thus improved.

Sometimes the population being considered—whether a whole population or a sampled one—is referred to as the *denominator*. Not all denominators need to be based on the practice population, nor on a subset of the practice population characterised by the presence of a particular disease or other characteristic. It can sometimes be useful to make measurements based on a series of consultations; for example, in attempting an audit of the care of children with cough, or of adults with back pain, the practice may monitor a sequence of consultations. Here it is important to include all the events in the series. Much can be learnt from, say, 50 consecutive consultations for a particular condition or complaint. By insisting that the denominator is made up of *consecutive* events, the practice may be able to generalise from the findings. If the auditor departs from this discipline—for example, by excluding the patients seen on Wednesdays or Fridays because the practice is particularly busy or understaffed on those days—the denominator can no longer be relied upon as being unbiased, and therefore the "findings" can have little relevance.

The individual case

A quite different approach to audit is based not on the measurement of populations or of series of events but on the evaluation of *individual significant events*. Examples from clinical medicine would include an audit of sudden or unexpected deaths, emergency admissions to hospital, suicide attempts, episodes of coronary thrombosis or stroke, newly registered blindness, episodes of iatrogenic illness, and mishaps. Examples from the organisation of the practice would include such matters as: the failure to visit the patient at home after a request for a visit had been accepted; a failure to despatch letters or to file them, or to take action on them; failure to deliver urgent messages; breakdown of relationships between members of the practice team; breaches of confidentiality; and so on.

The study of individual cases in an attempt to learn from mistakes and to experiment with new methods gave rise to what we now call the clinicopathological conference. This form of medical audit, with its basis in the postmortem room, has transformed the quality of clinical care in the hospital setting. A variety of clinicians, medical scientists, and others involved in the care of the patient critically examine their own performance and seek to learn from their own mistakes.

General practice has, in fact, developed a different but very strong tradition of case discussion, based on small groups. This teaching method has a central place in contemporary vocational training. Balint[10] seminars were perhaps the first and in many ways are still the most rigorous example of this method. Although the Balint approach is primarily concerned with the quality of the relationship between doctor and patient, developments over the past two decades have ensured that the physical components of the diagnosis and treatment, no less than the psychological and the social, have become subject to the same critical analysis. Although rarely described in these terms, Balint seminars and contemporary small group case discussions are among the most successful examples of medical audit in general practice in the United Kingdom. What may be missing is the recognition that these activities are a form of medical audit. They are, however, time consuming, their internal discipline is hard and takes time to learn, and the groups themselves need years rather than months to ensure that real learning and substantial change are taking place.

The audit of individual cases is likely to reveal two sources of error in the practice, knowledge of which can be invaluable. First, *case specific* errors can be detected. The medication for a chronic condition may have been inappropriate, or incompatible drugs may have been used. It may be discovered that there has been no expert evaluation of the retina of a diabetic patient over a period of years. Second, there may also have been *generic* errors, which point to the need to look at the organisation of the practice: letters and reports may have been incorrectly filed; no action may have been taken on an abnormal laboratory finding, when this had been intended.

Finally, the audit of individual cases should not be confined to the sort of critical events described above. An important technique that was first developed in Balint groups, and much used now in case discussion groups, is that of *random case analysis*. If this is to be successful those engaged in the audit must commit themselves to sticking strictly to the rules of the engagement. The group may decide in advance the case to be discussed—for example, the third patient to be seen next Tuesday morning. It is of no account that the third patient on that Tuesday only wants to check something on a previously issued certificate, or is deaf and unable to communicate properly, or has arrived in the consulting room by mistake, intending to see the nurse. The doctor whose case has to be audited must commit him- or herself to reporting that case and offer no excuse, however plausible, for choosing any other.

The ethos of medical audit

Modern general practice demands far more from the general practitioner than sound clinical practice. It demands the energetic management of a health service in miniature. With the advent of fundholding general practice, the scope of this management will become wider than previous experience has prepared us for, and the boundaries of the general practitioner's managerial responsibilities may eventually extend into many aspects of the specialist care of his or her patients in hospital.

Sound management, a prerequisite for the good quality of patient care, must be based on a clear vision of the intentions of the practice, an estimate of the size of, and the necessary resources for, the tasks to be undertaken, and a constant monitoring of performance against plans. The tools for this work, in essence the information and communication systems of the practice, are described elsewhere.

The concepts and techniques of medical audit are thus revealed as central to two linked tasks of general practice: solving clinical problems and managing the organisation. There is, however, a third task that medical audit must address and serve. General practice is not only a biotechnical enterprise and a managerial challenge, it is also a moral endeavour. The medicine of general practice is much concerned with optimising the resources of the individual, biological and psychological, spiritual and social, to cope with life's challenges and vicissitudes. It is concerned to represent the biotechnical possibilities of diagnosis and treatment on a human scale. It is concerned not with the fashionable—and perhaps fictional—battle between autonomy and dependency in the relationship between doctor and patient, but with a more subtle coming to an understanding with the patient about what he or she wants, needs, and is capable of achieving.

Part of this ethos is expressed in an appropriate openness between doctor and patient, and the new manifestation of this has been the growing interest in the accountability of the practice to the patients that it serves. The results of medical audit may thus in the future be reported not only to the practice personnel as a contribution to their professional development and the management of the practice but to the patients of the practice as a contribution to their own growing participation and personal responsibilities.

1 McIntyre N, Popper H. The critical attitude in medicine: the need for a new ethics. *BMJ* 1983;**287**:1919–23.
2 Berwick DM. Continuous improvement as an ideal in health care. *N Engl J Med* 1989;**320**:53–6.
3 Montagu A. Anthropology and medical education. *JAMA* 1963;**183**: 577.
4 McCormick J. Cervical smears: a questionable practice. *Lancet* 1989; **ii**:207–9.
5 Donabedian A. *Exploration in quality assessment and monitoring.* Vol 1. Ann Arbor: Health Administration Press, 1980.
6 Irvine D. *Teaching practices.* London: Royal College of General Practitioners, 1972. (Report from general practice No 15.)
7 Burke P. Otitis media: is medical management an option? *J R Coll Gen Pract* 1989;**39**:377–82.

8 Howie JGR, Porter AMD, Forbes JF. Quality and the use of time in general practice: widening the discussion. *BMJ* 1989;**298**:1008–10.

9 Hart JT. *Hypertension*. London and Edinburgh: Churchill Livingstone, 1980.

10 Balint M. *The doctor, his patient and the illness*. London: Tavistock, 1957.

2 Standards

MARSHALL MARINKER

I began the previous chapter with a reference to science. This was in recognition of the fact that medical audit is nothing less than an attempt to apply scientific method to the quest for quality. Scientific method demands that the terms we use be clearly defined. For this reason science, wherever possible, is discussed and communicated in an invented language of clearly defined symbols. In real language the word "mercurial" carries associations with a god, a planet, a metal, and a medicine. The *Oxford English Dictionary* gives such meanings as eloquence, ingenuity, aptitude for commerce, volatility, sprightliness, and ready wit.

In the language of chemistry the symbol Hg signifies one thing and one thing only: it describes a silver–white metallic element with a specific atomic number and mass. To define a word for the purposes of scientific endeavour we have to diminish its meanings. This is true of the most commonly used term in the lexicon of medical audit and quality assurance. That word is "standard." In living language the word carries associations with a flag or pennant, a stick or post, and a tree. It carries such meanings as basic, average, unimaginative, usual, measured, uniform, conforming, traditional, authoritative, desired, and excellent.

For the purposes of this book I shall define a *standard* as the performance the auditors have set themselves to achieve. In much of the literature on audit the word is given a more limited and specific definition—to denote the quantity of a particular component of audit. This can be confusing, and here we shall use the term "target" for this more specific purpose.

Tracers

Before standards can be set decisions have to be taken about the aspects of the practice that are to be considered for standard setting. Medical audit cannot address every aspect of the practice's work, the whole range of clinical conditions, the whole age range, or every aspect of the practice's organisation. In the previous chapter reference was made to the principle of economy of effort. The aim of medical audit must be to achieve the greatest benefit in terms of improved patient care for the most modest expenditure of resources—time, money, and personnel. The chosen audit should therefore not only be capable of giving information about the particular aspect of care under scrutiny but, if possible, should throw light on more general aspects of the care given by each doctor, or by the practice as a whole. These subjects of medical audit, chosen for their ability to reveal many aspects of the practice's performance, are known as *tracer conditions*. To sample a whole range of practice activities it is necessary to create some sort of framework so that different tracers can be selected to reflect the practice as a whole.

Kessner *et al*[1] suggested using at least two tracer conditions that were relevant to both sexes and to four broad age groups, and that a useful tracer should meet the following criteria:

1 A tracer should have a definite functional impact. By this I believe the authors mean that conditions that are not amenable to treatment, or that cause only negligible impairment, are unlikely to give useful information about the performance of the service being audited. A condition such as pityriasis rosea, which is self limiting and for which there is no specific treatment, would make a poor tracer.
2 A tracer should be well defined and easy to diagnose. Clearly hypertension would be well qualified. Depression, in contrast, because the diagnostic criteria are known to be much more elusive in general practice than they appear to be on the pages of psychiatric textbooks, might not qualify. If depression were chosen as a tracer a criterion such as the score on a well validated depression inventory rather than a diagnosis based solely on clinical judgment might be acceptable.
3 The prevalence rate should be high enough to permit the collection of adequate data from the population sample. In general practice an audit of the management of all those patients

17

with Crohn's disease would be inappropriate. The number of expected cases in a practice of average size would be too small. On the other hand, it would be perfectly possible to carry out a confidential inquiry into the care of an individual patient with Crohn's disease.

4 The natural history of the tracer condition should vary with the utilisation and effectiveness of medical care. Epilepsy and asthma would qualify well. Multiple sclerosis would not.

5 The techniques of medical management of the condition should be well defined for at least one of the following: prevention, diagnosis, treatment, or rehabilitation. Although this may be the easiest of Kessner's desiderata to satisfy, it should be remembered that Kessner requires all six of his desiderata if a tracer is to be regarded as really useful.

6 The effect of non-medical factors on the tracer should be understood. In general practice there is a need to take heed of the socioeconomic environment in which the audit is being carried out. Socioeconomic factors have the most profound effect not only on the prevalence of many diseases but on such factors as the decision to seek help, the natural history of the disease, compliance with treatment, and, even in the National Health Service, the availability of health care resources. A failure to appreciate the impact of these factors on health and health care results in the creation of quite unrealistic expectations.

Performance indicators

The concept of performance indicators is closely related to that of tracers. The word "tracer" refers to the condition that is to be considered. The term "performance indicators" refers to the tasks which are carried out by the health care workers involved. Maxwell[2] argued that health services should be assessed in at least six dimensions: relevance to need, ease of access, effectiveness, fairness, social acceptability, and efficiency and cost. The creative management of general practices in the future will undoubtedly demand that attention to be paid to all these six categories.

Best[3] identifies three criteria that validate a performance indicator. Firstly, the indicator must in some way be calibrated: ". . . this will usually mean that some measure of output will be expressed in relation to the input or inputs required to produce that output." Secondly, the indicator must be subject to unambiguous interpretation. Thirdly, changes in the indicator must be subject to influence by those whose performance is being judged. It would simply be dispiriting to identify need for change in a positive direction without either the authority or the means to bring about such change.

Monitoring the practice's repeat prescription system would seem to fulfil all three of Best's criteria. Firstly, a system that controlled the quantities and frequencies of repeat prescriptions, permitted a review of duration and dosage, and checked for pharmacologically incompatible regimens would clearly have a direct relationship to "output." Secondly, the detection of inappropriate prescribing, or of failure of compliance with an important continuing medication, might be thought to be fairly unambiguous in interpretation. Thirdly, changes in the indicator would certainly be within the capacity and control of those whose performance was being assessed.

In contrast, the monitoring of rates of referral to hospital would not fulfil all these important criteria. Although movement in the indicator would certainly be subject to influence by the doctor whose performance is being judged, it would be quite impossible to calibrate the performance, still less to interpret movements towards more or fewer referrals as in any way indicating improvements or deteriorations in the quality of care. There is as yet no research[4] that permits us to say that high, low, or mean rates of referral can be judged in terms of the appropriateness and quality of the doctor's referral practices.

The four chapters covering, respectively, chronic conditions, acute conditions, clinically significant events, and auditing practice management suggest a framework for selecting tracers. Clearly it is important that tracers be selected from at least each of the four major categories (or chapter headings) that we suggest. Which conditions are selected and how frequently there is a change of condition within each category are matters for practice policy. But practical considerations, the need to use limited resources for medical audit to best effect, suggest that practices should at any one time be economical in their choice of things to be audited.

Examples

As an example of the audit of patients with *chronic conditions* an audit of patients with diabetes mellitus will throw light on the practice's approach to the diagnosis, management, and monitoring of other chronic conditions. An audit of patients with schizophrenia will throw light on the management of psychiatric illness in a largely young adult population. An audit of palliative care will throw light not only on the practice's approach to the technical problems of therapeutics but also on the care of a more elderly population, on the approach to teamwork, and support for informal carers.

By the same token the choice of *acute conditions* to be monitored can also focus attention on particular age groups, or on particular aspects of the practice's performance. An audit of heart failure will focus on clinical and pharmacological skills in the care of older people. An audit of upper respiratory tract infection will focus on communication and health education skills in the care of young people and on the relationship of doctor, parent, and child.

The organisation of the practice can also be subjected to audit. Audits here might include: the response of staff to medical emergencies; an audit of the record system and quality of the notes; an audit of the repeat prescription system; laboratory and imaging investigations; and referral letters to hospital consultants. All of this is predicated on the notion that criteria will be recognised, against which performance can be assessed.

An anatomy of standards

Having selected a tracer, the auditors next have to decide on a number of relevant *criteria* which can be measured. Criteria are components of the tracer condition that are thought to be relevant to the performance of the doctor or the practice. In the case of hypertension, for example, good criteria might include the percentage of discovered hypertensive patients in the adult population, the medications employed, and measurements of blood pressure after treatment.

A *standard* is created when these criteria are given certain quantitative or qualitative characteristics. Such standards in fact serve as *targets* and the reason for preferring this term is given at the beginning of this chapter. Our knowledge of the incidence of moderate to severe hypertension in an adult population, corrected for its age/sex structure, permits the practice to predict the approximate percentage of "cases" which could be found by total successful screening. The actual number of cases found after five years of opportunistic screening—that is, monitoring the blood pressure of all adults who present to the practice for no matter what clinical problem—can then be compared with this "expected" figure, so that some estimate can be made of the efficiency of the practice's screening programme. Other criteria may be used and targets may be agreed that will reflect other aspects of the care of hypertensive patients. What levels of blood pressure control were achieved? To what extent did the medication actually used comply with the range of drugs that the practice had agreed to employ?

A *protocol* for diagnosis or treatment is a statement about optimum performance. In the case of diagnosis the practice may wish to stipulate a number of necessary preconditions that must be met to establish the diagnosis. For example, in the case of hypertension the practice may demand that the blood pressure be taken on more than one occasion; it may specify whether the patient is sitting or standing; it may rely on measures of diastolic or systolic pressure, or both; it may decide on the highest readings, or the lowest readings, or the mean of all the readings. The literature on hypertension is unhelpfully replete with advice on this, much of it contradictory. Most general practices will resist the temptation to make a thorough search of the literature and a critical review of it. For the purposes of clinical audit there is often a consensus view that serves as a basis for standard setting. How is this consensus view formed?

Quite often this view begins with the opinions of specialists in a particular field, based on a mixture of their clinical experience and their interpretation of the literature. One of the major strengths of medical audit is that it compels the auditors to look with fresh eyes at received clinical wisdom. It is important to remember that for the most part textbook descriptions of disease, and textbook recommendations for treatment, are based on the experience of secondary medical care—on the experience of specialists who mostly see only those patients referred to them by general practitioners. The textbook picture is therefore both incomplete and potentially misleading. If standards are to be set for general practice they must be set in general practice. Some sort of dialogue will then be necessary not only among the general practitioners in partnership who wish to audit their own work but between general practitioners and the relevant specialists concerned. Such discussions and negotiations are described in the chapter on group work.

Protocols may take many forms. They may consist of questions to be answered, actions to be carried out, or choices to be made.

Sometimes a protocol is given the form of an *algorithm*, which is a graphic display of binary logic. These algorithms, if they are to reflect the wide range of possibilities and choices that are encountered in practice, can sometimes appear rambling and confusing. This is because the algorithm depicts not the way in which the doctor thinks but rather the way in which the computer has been taught to process. Clearly I dislike them.

Standards that are derived from textbook and specialist sources, even when mediated by general practice experience, are described as *ideal* or *normative*. The danger here is that these so called ideal standards may be unrealistic, and may sometimes be actually damaging. Standards can be unrealistic if they do not take into account the true prevalence and incidence of events in general practice. In past decades some of the protocols for optimum diagnosis and treatment in the United States of America begin to resemble the aggregated small print of major specialist textbooks written up as a brief for the defence in a law suit. Protocols in general practice should reflect the tasks of general practice. The task of the specialist[5] is to reduce uncertainty, to pursue possibility, and to marginalise error. The task of the general practitioner is to accept uncertainty, to explore probability, and to marginalise danger. General practice protocols should reflect general practice realities.

The general practitioner has to consider what uncertainties it is safe to tolerate: when a child presents with acute pain in an ear obscured by wax; when he is consulted by a young woman who has unaccountably stumbled and fallen for a third time in a year; or when he considers what to do next for a middle aged woman whose indigestion persists in spite of alkali mixtures and cimetidine. What probabilities does he need to explore: when an adolescent girl loses weight; when an octogenarian complains of giddiness on getting out of bed; when a young wife tells her doctor that her husband probably needs a good physical checkup? What dangers must be marginalised: when a child presents with high fever; when a young woman presents with colicky abdominal pain; when an elderly widow comes to tell her doctor that her pet dog has had to be put down?

The clinical competencies of general practice are derived from values that have all but disappeared in late twentieth century medicine. What society values in our times is excellence in specialism: this demands a deep and penetrating understanding of a restricted field of endeavour, with an emphasis on technical skills, convergent thinking, rationality, and the explicit.

Excellence in generalism is quite different. It is characterised by: a superficial grasp of a very wide field of endeavour; problem solving that is horizontal rather than vertical; thinking that is as much convergent as divergent; skills that are not so much technical as interactive; room not only for the rational and the explicit but also for the intuitive and the implicit.

The United Kingdom is both a multiracial and a multicultural society. Members of ethnic minorities exhibit particular patterns of morbidity, including morbidities that may be associated with the effects of immigration itself, and these may be manifest in the families of immigrants over more than one generation. Further, populations of ethnic minorities have their own particular social needs, health beliefs, expectations of medical care, and many other factors that can affect health, health care, and the way in which the practices that serve them can perform. As a result of these factors, standard setting must be carried out with sensitivity to these important local variables. It is also worth recalling that even within the host or majority culture there may be local variables such as the socioeconomic structure of the practice population, the availability of health care resources, and so on.

When a protocol reflects these general practice realities the standards are described as *pragmatic*. The danger here is that the term, indeed the very idea, can be used as an alibi for poor or unacceptable standards. This does not have to be so. Pragmatic standards must above all be safe: that is to say they must fully explore probability and maximally marginalise danger.

Confidential inquiries

Perhaps the standards of care in which the doctor can have most trust are those that emerge from the search for avoidable errors in his or her own clinical work. I described this approach to the individual case in the preceding chapter. A group undertaking such a confidential inquiry into an individual significant event needs to pay attention to a number of issues in the quest for better standards. Six essential steps may be recalled by the use of the acronym REPOSE.

First, the *reason* for the inquiry shoud be clearly stated. For example, a woman may have become pregnant while taking an

23

oral contraceptive. It is discovered that she has also taken another prescribed medicine—an antibiotic which has possibly interfered with the contraceptive action of the pill. Next, the *evidence* needs to be presented. What evidence is there in the research literature of interaction between the pill and other medication? Partnerships will need to become confident in the critical reading of research evidence, not least in assessing the size of risk and the implications for clinical decision making in general practice. These considerations will result in the formulation of a *policy*. Experience, however, suggests that care must be taken to ensure that all those who will be involved in pursuing this policy understand it, agree with it, and are motivated to carry it out. This means that the audit group must ensure that those involved have a sense of *ownership* of this policy. When this has been done a *system* can be devised to ensure that the policy is adhered to—for example, the medical records of all women known to be taking oral contraceptives can, following consultation, be reviewed by the practice nurse to note compliance. Last, the audit group can agree to make *inquiry* at a given interval to ensure that compliance with the policy has been achieved. Only by attention to all these steps can the audit group repose trust in the validity of the standards that follow from such an exercise.

Norms

Finally, standards may be derived not from research or clinical opinion or local negotiation but rather from a belief in the inherent worth or statistical averages or *norms*. The longest established medical audit in British general practice, that of prescribing, is based on such a belief. Doctors are provided with statistics about their own prescribing, and are given as reference points the prescribing averages for their partnership, their locality, and their region. These norms then become either implicit targets or, sometimes, implicit ceilings. No attempt is made to correlate the level of prescribing, in terms of the number of prescriptions issued or the average cost of prescriptions, with the quality of care. There is an undeclared consensus, or perhaps a conspiracy, to equate these norms with virtue.

The same would not be true if the Department of Health sought to apply such norms to judgments about rates of referral to hospital. In one major study[6] the difference in referral rates between doctors in the top and bottom quintiles of the study population was fourfold. Despite such large disparities, the researchers were unable to draw any conclusions linking rates of referral to the quality of care.

Judgments

Standards are sometimes referred to as *explicit* and *implicit*. Any standard that is to be applied to a population must be explicit—that is to say, it must be stated clearly and unambiguously, and wherever possible quantified. Difficulties arise, however, when we try to apply unambiguous explicit standards to individual cases—for example, in confidential inquiries or in sampling individual case notes where the audit reveals a departure from the standards set. Here judgments can only be made in relation to the clinical experience and values of the auditors. The auditors have to ask the questions:

"What would we ourselves have done in these circumstances?"
"What reasonable steps might have been taken?"
"What external factors made it difficult or impossible to adhere to the agreed procotol?"

Sometimes it is possible to make explicit what might otherwise appear to be entirely implicit judgments. For example, in judging the quality of case discussions, I suggested the following catechism:[7]

- Has the problem been effectively identified?
- Has the problem been resolved in the shortest possible time?
- Has the number of problem solving steps been reduced to a minimum consonant with safety?
- Has the simplest technology been employed?
- Has the optimum medication been selected and monitored?
- Has the management caused the minimum harm or risk of harm to the patient?
- Has there been optimum use of health care personnel?
- Have self care and family care been fully mobilised?
- What realistic criteria of success were adopted, and were they achieved?

One of the most commonly voiced objections to medical audit is that it is impossible to apply explicit standards (applicable to

25

populations) to the individual case. This objection is valid if such explicit standards are insensitively applied without recourse to implicit judgment. In judging an individual case explicit protocols should be used to pose questions about the clinical care. They must not be used simply to pass arbitrary judgments about what is good or bad.

Conclusion

The search for standards begins with some sensible and pragmatic questions about what we are trying to achieve. A group of doctors may begin with the question, "Why not look at how we treat depression?" They will be driven to ask, "How often do we make the diagnosis now, and what do we do about it?" Next they may ask, "How does my performance compare with that of others and is there anything that I can learn from this comparison?" Before too long, however, other questions suggest themselves: "What do we mean by the term 'depression'?" and then "What is the received wisdom about this, and where is the evidence?"

Setting standards is the prerequisite of good management; monitoring and achieving them are the goals of good management. But this alone is not enough. I began this chapter by considering the meanings that have attached themselves to the word. The word "standard" carries with it shades of authority, certainty, and permanence. But this is not the essence of clinical science. The search for standards demands a constant reconsideration of what we know, how we know it, and how we understand it. The search for standards is the purpose of medical audit. In this sense medical audit becomes the ultimate refresher course, in every meaning of that term.

1 Kessner DM, Kalk CE, Singer J. Assessing health quality—the case for tracers. *N Engl J Med* 1977;**288**:189–94.
2 Maxwell RJ. Quality assessment in health. *BMJ* 1984;**288**:1470–2.
3 Best GA. Performance indicators: a precautionary tale for unit managers. In: Wickings HI, ed, *Effective unit management.* King Edward's Hospital Fund for London, 1983:62–83.
4 Marinker M, Wilkin D, Metcalfe D. Referral to hospital: can we do better? *BMJ* 1988;**297**:461–4.

5 Marinker M. *Greening the White Paper.* London: Social Market Foundation, 1989.
6 Wilkin D, Smith AG. Variations in general practitioner's referral rates to consultants. *J R Coll Gen Pract* 1987;**37**:350–3.
7 Marinker M. Case discussion. In: Cormack J, Marinker M, Morrell D, eds, *Teaching general practice.* London: Kluwer, 1981:105–11.

3 How to begin

MICHAEL DRURY, BILL STYLES

The term "medical audit" provokes a wide variety of responses among those who are called upon to take part. This ranges from the perception that it is another managerial activity that has been forced on a reluctant medical profession and that impedes clinical work, to the views of those who see it as an essential component in the pursuit of high clinical standards and cost effective medical care. We belong unashamedly to the second group but we recognise that the alternative view requires us to spell out what we see as the advantages to be gained by a practice's participation in audit.

The term "audit," with its undertones of finance and being called to account, also has the capacity to produce negative feelings in people who regard themselves as "giving" a service to patients in need. Yet it is likely that all those in the practice are already concerned with improving aspects of their work, and such improvement is the underlying purpose of medical audit. It can make important contributions to the further education and professional development of every member of the practice team, and it can make fundamental contributions to improving the quality of patient care. These are its essential benefits, and whatever arrangements are made for audit within a practice they must be directed towards these purposes. Although audit can be developed as an instrument of accountability, its main goals must relate to education and to standards of patient care.[1] Its success in these areas will depend upon the active participation of those practice members who together have agreed to review their own performance and the quality of their work. Among the benefits to be derived from audit there is the capacity to lessen the possibility of mistakes occurring in clinic work, to remove annoyance from administrative delay, and to counter potential patient dissatisfaction with the quality of service that is offered. If these seem rather negative attributes then they may expressed as improving clinical care, improving efficiency, and promoting relationships.

For those requiring a more practical demonstration of the relevance of audit to everyday activity before they will invest time and trouble, we need look no further than three examples of the normal frustrations experienced by any member of a practice team:

1 Patients complain to the practice manager about their inability to get through on the telephone at certain times of the day. An audit of the use of the telephone can reveal the times when this occurs, the nature of the telephone calls, the systems for answering incoming calls, the nature of outgoing calls, and the reasons why telephone lines may be blocked at these times. The end result could be a measurable lessening of delay, better patient access, a change in patterns of demand, and possibly even lower telephone bills.

2 Much time and effort is expended in setting up clinics in shared asthma care. Doctors and nurses continue to wonder about the benefits of this activity to patients. An audit may show levels of patient satisfaction with the system; it may show the effect on some measures of outcome, such as drug consumption, acute attacks of asthma, or time off school or work. It will almost certainly show a dearth of data about patients which could have an important bearing on prescribing costs, work load, and patient well being.

3 The practice may be aware that many patients who return for the results of investigations have to be told that they are not yet available. An audit may identify the causes of delay and how these can be lessened. It may also begin to reveal wide variations in demand for investigations among the partners in a practice and this could stimulate other audit activities.

It is probable that many members of the practice team have already been involved with audit procedures through simple projects undertaken within the practice, or by participating when visiting other practices, or through trainer selection procedures. The selection of general practitioner trainers on the basis of agreed regional criteria is one of the commonest exercises in medical audit in general practice. Nevertheless, the prospect of embarking on

29

medical audit in a more systematic and organised way will cause concern within every practice. These concerns will have to be addressed if future activities are not to be prejudiced by indifference or even by hostility within the practice team.

Possible obstacles and pitfalls

There will be a number of obstacles and pitfalls in the early stages. Therefore good groundwork at this point will prevent difficulties later on. Firstly, it is essential that everyone in the practice is briefed about the nature and the objectives of audit. Although it is possible to do this at a large practice meeting involving all staff, it is probably better to begin with a series of small meetings when the principles are still being debated. It is essential that the partners in the practice should be clear about the purpose of audit and committed to future activities involving it, and so, too, must all members of the practice staff be clear. It is inevitable that some members of the group will be defensive, feeling that they do not have the necessary ability for work with audit. Others may have major reservations and misconceptions about what audit is and what purpose it serves. All these difficulties must be resolved early on, otherwise they will soon become the focus for discontent. People will be anxious about the time involved and will fear the intrusion of audit activities into what, for many, is already a busy working schedule. Some anxieties about time may reflect the doubts that members of the practice might have about their abilities to participate in such work and all this has to be explored in a sensitive way. Before long some will begin to show enthusiasm for the suggestion of being involved in audit projects and soon a series of proposals will begin to emerge. The next difficulty will be in considering everyone's different priorities so that a starting point can be determined.

At this stage it is worth reviewing once more the overall benefits of audit and why the practice is undertaking it. What does the practice team hope to learn from this work? How will it help each of the members in continuing education and professional development? How will it lead to more efficient practice management and to the more appropriate use of time and other practice resources? How will it contribute to more effective care and, in this way, benefit the patients in the practice? The practice must be clear from the start how the results of the audit exercise will be used.

Emphasis must be laid on the confidential nature of the work and the fact that it is designed to lead to improvements in the services of the practice through modification in practice routines and that most certainly it will not be linked to sanctions and to punishment of practice members. In the early stages most practices are content to limit the results of their audit activities to the members of the practice. As confidence and trust develop some are prepared to share their results and to compare them with other local practices, sometimes under the umbrella of the Medical Audit Advisory Group (MAAG), of local medical committees, and of local faculties of the Royal College of General Practitioners.

Agreement within the practice team

Once the partners have agreed in general terms the purposes of the audit and how it will be undertaken, the broad concept should be discussed with the other members of the practice team and particularly with the practice manager, who will have a key role in designing and running systems that are introduced. The reservations and concerns that may already have been expressed and explored with the partners will undoubtedly be shared by the other members of the team. Once again, it is important to understand these fears and to ensure that each member of the practice understands the overall purpose of the audit exercises that are proposed.

Clinical audits on the care of specific conditions will almost certainly involve the nurses in the practice, whereas audits of the administrative procedures, such as appointment systems, hospital referrals, and so on, will be the concern of the practice receptionists and secretaries.

Sooner or later, for any audit, all practice staff will become involved so that it is important from the outset to have all members committed and convinced of the merit of the work that is proposed.

Everyone must be convinced of the value of the audit to them and their aspirations for patients. Early discussions will provide opportunities for practice staff to share their overall vision of the work of the practice. It will be important to focus on the area of work of each of them and to listen to their views. The cost of audit to them will take time and to people who already consider

31

themselves busy this may seem to be yet another "last straw." A fear of lack of time will be a reasonable anxiety: it is often the excuse that some will use to hide from the threat that audit will expose deficiencies in their work. Such fears must be clearly understood by those proposing involvement in audit and the sensitive handling of such issues is vital if progress is to be made.

Most of us will have different agendas for this exercise and people will need to have an opportunity to put their priorities forward and to recognise that, as audit becomes a continuing programme, they will be able to organise their own activities. In any case, once each understands that audit is essentially educational he or she will soon realise that all of us learn from every audit. It is clearly important, however, that from the start subjects are chosen that are generally relevant to the care of patients and to the training of practice staff.

Time and enthusiasm are precious commodities that must not be squandered. The aims of audit tasks must therefore be realistic and the tasks should be capable of completion. Picking a subject for which it is too difficult to collect and analyse the data, or one for which it would be impossible to implement the necessary changes that it highlights, would be a bad start. It is much better to agree a relatively simple, albeit important and relevant objective, from which a result can be obtained before enthusiasm wanes. As people's confidence builds up it is possible to shift towards more esoteric and complex areas. It is much easier to bear failure at a later stage when successes have already been obtained; early failures can halt the programme.

What to audit

Having agreed to become involved in audit, the practice team must then decide on the activity to be studied. This can be an analysis of a clinical aspect of the practice's work or a review of one of the non-clinical systems that supports it. An example of the latter might be to review the efficiency of the practice's appointment system or the arrangements for access to out of hours care.

Having agreed the practice activity to be studied, the members of the practice team must then determine what they are trying to achieve in this particular area. The results of the audit will then indicate how successful the practice is in reaching its previously agreed targets. These results will form the basis upon which the practice will decide how to improve its performance in this particular area. A rerun of audit at a later date will then demonstrate how successful or otherwise the practice has been in bringing about the improvements that the first audit had suggested were necessary.

In the language of medical audit the practice will have decided the criteria for the audit activity—that is, the elements to be studied within the practice—as well as the standards that will operate. Standards are explicit statements that indicate precisely what the practice has agreed are the acceptable levels of performance for which it is aiming. Agreeing standards can be difficult: they should be realistic and achievable while being at a level the practice has yet to attain.

Type of audit: quantitative or qualitative?

Having decided the area of activity for audit, the practice must then agree how the audit will be undertaken. In general terms there are two types of audit. The first depends upon the collection and analysis of data about a large number of patients or events. The second does not have such a quantitative basis and is based on the review of the time leading up to a significant or critical event. Such an event might be the unexpected death of a patient, the emergency admission of an asthmatic child to hospital, a case of measles, a young woman with carcinoma of the cervix, or the onset of blindness in a diabetic patient. Such a qualitative audit would involve all members of the practice team associated with the patient and its success would depend considerably on the accuracy of practice records.

The more quantitative type of medical audit depends on meticulous forward planning—on agreeing the activity to be reviewed and the people who will be involved, together with the data that will be collected and analysed. There is a tendency to opt for activities that are easily measurable. Whereas this is certainly to be recommended for a practice that is becoming involved in audit for the first time, it must be recognised that easily measurable aspects of a practice's work are not necessarily the best measures of its overall quality of care. Easily measurable activities include a practice's preventive services—for example, the childhood immunisation rates or cervical cytology.

The review of the care of patients with chronic disease lends itself readily to quantitative medical audit. An essential early step

33

is to agree a practice protocol for the care of the chronic disease being studied. Many practices have found the protocols for chronic conditions that have been prepared by the Royal College of General Practitioners to be good starting points for the generation of their practice's own standards and procedures. Other practice activities that are readily measurable include prescribing and the efficiency of the practice's appointment system.

Agreeing criteria and standards

Having determined the practice activity to be reviewed, the next step is to decide the objectives that the practice works towards. Criteria are those elements of care that will be counted or measured to determine the quality. The standards will represent the measurements that the practice has agreed will reflect an acceptable level of care. Value judgments are involved in determining both of these and they will reflect the views of individuals in the team, as well as the current objectives of the general medical care system, which will usually be based on the evidence of scientific research.

The question that the members of the practice must be able to answer at this early stage is: "What are we trying to achieve through this particular activity?" Linked to this will be concerns about a particular practice activity—clinical or organisational. They will then agree the purpose of the audit that they are embarking on. The next step will be to measure the practice's overall level of performance against the standards (objectives) that they have agreed, which are based on the views and evidence that they have collected. These will be linked to the aims of the practice for the activity being studied, particularly to the processes for achieving these aims and to the outcomes.

Standards can be generated in either of two ways: through a review of the medical literature on the subject and an analysis of the perceived wisdom at that time, *or* by collecting data about the practice's present level of performance and then agreeing future targets from the information that these will yield.

On some occasions the members of a practice may agree standards based on information obtained in both these ways.

The information generated from the research literature and from the practice itself will then form the basis for discussion so that agreed standards of care can be determined by all those involved in the audit exercise. These standards will then form the basis of the exercise itself.

Additional information is collected and can be obtained from the Family Health Services Authority or the Health Board (for example, about items of service activities) or from the Prescription Pricing Authority. Such information can be of great help in auditing certain practice activities. In general, however, the collection of data by the practice itself has much to commend it, because the information derived from it would be of greater accuracy than that obtained from sources outside the practice.

Age/sex register

Although some Family Health Service Authorities will provide age/sex registers free of charge, they are still maintained by only a minority of practices and only used by a proportion of the practices that have them. They have been thought by some doctors to be research tools. Although they are a key feature for research in general practice, they can contribute much to the efficient management of the practice and will be essential if the practice wishes to develop a full range of medical audit exercises; for example, it is not possible to know which 12 year old girls in the practice are immunised against rubella unless the practice has a list that distinguishes that practice population by age and sex. This will be important for any practice that needs to know the proportion of preventive services it undertakes and if it wishes to maximise or check its income.

Until recently many practices have kept an age/sex register by means of a card index system listing males and females in groups by year of birth. These cards have been marked or tagged to indicate, say, which of the patients have had their blood pressure recorded within five years and which, more importantly, have not. It is immediately apparent how such a simple system can be used in audit. If, for example, the practice agrees that all patients between the ages of, say, 30 and 65 should have their blood pressure recorded every five years then it is possible by using a tagged age/sex card system to know for how many this has been achieved and how many will need to have their blood pressures measured to secure a 100% target. To undertake such a simple audit exercise would be almost impossible without a tagged age/sex register.

The development of computers within general practice makes it much easier to develop an age/sex register and to keep it up to date. The importance of updating the practice age/sex register should be emphasised; it must be as accurate as possible because it provides one of the most important denominator populations for medical audit in general practice, namely the registered patient list. There is much to be said for practice staff ensuring every quarter that the practice age/sex register is up to date by checking that all new patients who have registered in the previous three months are included in the register and that those who have left have had their names removed from it. There is also a considerable advantage in comparing at regular intervals the age/sex register held in the practice with that held by the family practitioner committee or health board.

There are many other uses for the age/sex register, particularly for simple practice management as a directory of names, addresses, and telephone numbers, and as a profile of the practice for planning purposes, especially when it includes details of social class and ethnic groups.

The morbidity index

The second source of denominators within a practice population is the morbidity index. This provides lists of the patients who have particular problems that interest the practice. A few hundred practices, and particularly those involved in the national morbidity survey and the weekly return services of the Royal College of General Practitioners, have developed complete morbidity recording. Every diagnosis made in these practices is classified according to a coded system and is listed under the appropriate heading. This enables the practice or researchers working with it to determine how many new diagnoses of a particular condition are made each year (the incidence of the problem) and how many patients are on the list with that problem (the prevalence of the problem). For example, a practice of 10 000 people may have 700 patients with asthma: so that the prevalence of asthma is 7%. Within the year only 20 new diagnoses of asthma may have been made, giving an incidence of 0·2%.

For most practices a more limited form of morbidity index will be appropriate. It will be for each practice to decide upon the medical conditions and special interests that it wishes included in its own index; for example, practices whose members wish to organise special sessions for the care of patients with asthma, diabetes, or hypertension will need accurate lists of all patients with these conditions so that they can monitor certain aspects of their care. Thus the morbidity index will be the starting point for determining the denominator population for audit of the quality of care of these patients.

Once the criteria for their care have been agreed, the patients with the condition being studied can be identified from the morbidity index and the medical records of each can then be reviewed to determine the extent to which the agreed standards for care have been applied. For example, are they being followed up at appropriate intervals? Is the information that was agreed to be essential being recorded properly? Is the control achieved, for example, of blood pressure levels and of blood sugar levels, measuring up to the agreed standards for good care?

Such data, acquired from the patient's individual medical record, are needed to monitor management against the practice's agreed standards. So, too, is a morbidity index to provide the denominator population.

The use of the computer in medical audit

Age/sex registers and morbidity indexes have been developed in practices for many years and, necessarily, have been kept in a manual way. The advent of the computer in general practice is rapidly changing this and makes the use of these registers and indexes much easier and quicker. The age/sex register of the practice must be included in any general practice computer program and this is so for most of the commonly used systems in general practice at the moment. Computers can print out lists and sublists of categories of patients and in this way they can contribute considerably to audit.

Most systems can produce the names and addresses of all children and different age groups and so allow the measuring, for example, of the proportion of children who have not been immunised and for whom special measures will need to be taken. Such information is essential for the proper management of the practice and for maximising its income. It also enables the practice to measure how close it is to achieving its agreed targets for immunisation performance, and in the light of this to plan how to improve its procedures and to work towards higher standards of preventive care for the children in the practice population. The next stage is to repeat the audit cycle by measuring the effect of the changes that have been made earlier to ensure that they have resulted in the improvements that were considered necessary.

As the practice moves to a more sophisticated system, with a computer terminal in every consulting room and a diagnosis recorded on computer at every consultation, a computer held morbidity index will be built up and its use as an instrument to audit disease categories will be further enhanced.

The prescribing of new or repeat prescriptions through the computer also enables it to provide information about further subgroups within the practice population and thereby provide a different range of denominators; for example, the number of women on the contraceptive pill, the number of men on antihypertensive drugs, and those on anticonvulsant or antiasthmatic medication are denominators of population that can provide the basis for further audit studies.

Qualitative audit

Most of the audit work that has been undertaken to date in general practice has been of a quantitative type. Many practices have enjoyed collecting and analysing information about subgroups of patients within the practice population. The computer is making such work easier and has added an impetus to this type of activity. Qualitative audit is not based on the analysis of numbers or on large subgroups of a practice population. Nevertheless, some find it more challenging intellectually than quantitative audit, for it gets closer to the caring aspect of practice and to examining the extent to which each patient's real needs are met. Through qualitative audit the social and psychological components of care can be more easily examined. Nevertheless, qualitative audit can be as rigorous as quantitative audit, provided that the criteria agreed have been carefully defined.

In essence, qualitative audit consists of reviewing the records of patients and analysing on an individual basis whether or not the quality of care has met the standards that have been agreed by the practice. An analysis of this kind is usually triggered by a significant or critical event, and practices should agree in advance the events that might lead to such a review of patient care. Hospital obstetricians have undertaken such work for many years through the review of perinatal deaths, a review that most obstetric units carry out on a regular basis.

In the obstetric system of audit every case is rigorously examined by the group of doctors involved, to see that everything that had been agreed previously has been done. Were all the tests that should have been carried out in the prenatal period done? Was the labour managed appropriately? Were the grieving relatives treated properly? Was the general practitioner informed quickly? Given enough cases, this work can be quantified, but its value lies in the careful review of each case so that action for improvement can be taken on the basis of one single review.

In general practice there is a series of events that can be reviewed in this way. Although some of these might include the death of patients, and particularly their sudden death, they may not all be based on such an outcome; for example, the emergency admission of a child with asthma to hospital could provide a worthwhile basis for the exercise. Others might include a young woman with diagnosed cervical cancer, or a request for termination of pregnancy, or a relapsed schizophrenic patient. The list is endless and careful selection is needed to ensure that the topic being audited is important, relevant, and capable of giving a reasonably quick answer that can lead to improvement.

Collaborative audit

As competence with medical audit grows within a practice its members will wish to share their experiences and compare their results with others. In some localities medical audit groups have been established in postgraduate medical centres and in some instances through the local faculty of the Royal College of General Practitioners. In these groups some presentations are made of audits undertaken in particular practices, but mostly general exercises are developed so that the same aspects of care can be compared between practices. On some occasions special data collection forms have been agreed so that comparisons can be made. Many have found this work stimulating and enjoyable and a potent way of encouraging progress. The importance of ensuring that the data can be analysed in a manner that permits comparisons between practices cannot be overstated. In particular, the denominator population between the practices must be the same and results must be expressed as comparable rates.

Audit at the interface between hospital and general practice

As audit techniques develop there will be opportunities for collaborative audit between those working in general practice and those in the hospital setting. There will be occasions when activities at the interface itself can be monitored—for example, the appropriateness of hospital referrals; the delay in outpatient appointments; the communication between general practitioners and hospital specialists; and the efficiency of procedures before discharge from hospital, particularly for elderly patients. There will also be opportunities to review together the care of patients with selected groups of chronic conditions and to compare the utilisation rates of laboratory and radiological facilities between hospital and general practice based colleagues.

Tracer conditions

It is not possible to audit every aspect of general practice or every medical condition seen within that setting. Some are easier to study than others, and these usually form the basis for tracer conditions. The assumption is made that the quality of care demonstrated for certain tracer conditions is a reasonably accurate measure of the quality provided for all the other illnesses dealt with in general practice.

The characteristics of a tracer condition are as follows:

- It should have a definite functional impact on those affected
- The condition should be well defined and easy to diagnose
- Its prevalence rate should be high to be able to provide adequate numbers for study
- Its natural history must be modified by suitable treatment
- Its management must be well defined in terms of prevention, diagnosis, treatment, or rehabilitation
- The effect of non-medical factors on the tracer condition should be understood.

Using these criteria many tracer conditions can be identified in general practice. These would include chronic conditions such as hypertension, diabetes mellitus, epilepsy, asthma, and thyroid disease, as well as more acute disorders such as otitis media and urinary tract infection. A practice's morbidity index, particularly if computerised, will readily provide populations of these patients for medical audit purposes.

Using the results of medical audit

It should be agreed at the outset who is responsible for analysing the data and preparing the results. It is essential that the results should be presented in writing to all those members of the practice team who have been involved in the exercise. There should be an opportunity at a suitable meeting for all involved to come together to consider the results and how they will be used.

Consideration should be given to the audit exercise itself. How effective has it been? Was the experience as unpleasant as some had thought it might be? How could it have been improved? Were the data that were collected appropriate and might there have been better ways of gathering the information? Were the standards that were agreed reasonable ones? Was the project well designed and relevant overall to the needs of the practice?

Then the results of the exercise must be considered. What lessons can be learnt from them? How much more effort is needed for the practice to reach its agreed standards? Who will be responsible for bringing about some of the changes that have been found to be necessary?

By the end of the audit exercise there should emerge a management plan for the future. This should identify clearly the people who will be responsible for its implementation so that the results of the project can be directed towards better quality patient care.

The audit cycle

The members of the practice must also consider when they will next repeat an audit in this particular area of practice activity. Then, on that occasion, the details for the next round of the audit cycle must be agreed and must take account of the many lessons learnt from the previous effort. In this way the effects of implementing the changes found by previous audit exercises can be measured and the overall success of the audit itself can be demonstrated for that particular activity. To undertake a single audit exercise within a given practice activity is fruitless. The strength of audit is its cyclical nature and the opportunity that it provides for measuring the effects of changes in practice routine which have been stimulated by previous audit procedures. Michael Sheldon[2] has demonstrated the five steps of medical audit, emphasising the importance of step 5, which is to repeat the audit exercise to find out whether or not the care of patients has improved as a result of previous efforts. Only by doing this can audit itself be audited.

Guidance and some warnings

It may help at this point to sum up the factors for success in medical audit. These are as follows:

- Agreement on the value of audit
- Agreement on the purpose of audit
- Taking account of the concerns of partners and practice staff (suspicion, lack of time, perceived lack of skills)
- Agreement on the practice activities to be studied
- Agreement on roles, especially for data collection, analysis, and reporting results
- Agreement on standards, based on a review of the literature and/ or present levels of practice activity
- Ensuring that the area of study is relevant
- Ensuring that data collection is easy, based on data already available within the practice
- Ensuring that the denominator population is well defined
- Ensuring that the condition studied is common in general practice
- Ensuring that the results can lead to the implementation of change
- Ensuring that the results are clearly expressed
- Ensuring that the results are considered
- Identifying those responsible for implementing the changes agreed to be necessary
- Agreement on a date for the rerun of an audit
- Completion of the audit cycle.

It may also help to give warnings about the problem areas to look for. These include the following:

- Information gathering in itself does not constitute audit: analysis is needed
- Agreement on standards is not easy and can cause difficulties
- Data collection can be laborious, particularly if it is not perceived as relevant and if it is not part of the normal practice routine
- Securing the involvement of all members of the practice
- Poor and impractical design of a project that requires excessive servicing will lead to problems
- The lack of a clear purpose for a project causes problems
- Poor practice records and no clear denominator population will cause failure.

Conclusion

Medical audit has now become an everyday practice activity. It is important to ensure that the time and effort spent produce good results, so that the practice can be managed more efficiently and so that the quality of care available to patients can be enhanced. Once overcome, the suspicion and resistance to audit shown by some doctors and practice staff will give way to enjoyment and enthusiasm as the relevance of audit work to the work of the practice becomes apparent. Its success will depend on maintaining the confidentiality of those involved and dealing sensitively with any concerns that are expressed by practice staff. Audit must never be seen as a punitive exercise, with punishment and sanctions. It must be developed as an important part of the quest for higher standards of patient care. The elements for success include practice records of high quality, age/sex registers, and morbidity indexes, as well as time when members of the practice can meet together to discuss this aspect of their work, to plan it carefully, to consider the results achieved, and to agree the changes in practice routine that may be found necessary.

1 Pendleton D, Schofield T, Marinker M. *In pursuit of quality—approaches to performance review in general practice.* London: Royal College of General Practitioners, 1986; Baker R. *Practice assessment and quality of care.* London: Royal College of General Practitioners, 1988. (Occasional

paper 39.) Watkins CJ. *The measurement of quality in general practitioner care.* London: Royal College of General Practitioners, 1981. (Occasional paper 15.)

2 Sheldon G. *Medical audit in general practice.* London: Royal College of General Practitioners, 1982. (Occasional paper 20.) (Butterworth Prize Essay 1981.)

4 Chronic conditions

COLIN WAINE

As the purpose of audit is to improve the quality of care of patients, those chronic conditions where appropriate intervention can materially benefit the patient, and where inappropriate intervention or failure to take appropriate action can harm the patient, provide excellent subjects for medical audit. Examples would include heart failure, postmyocardial infarction, epilepsy, eczema, and rheumatoid arthritis. In this chapter I give diabetes mellitus and asthma as examples.

Diabetes mellitus

Diabetes, one of the most prevalent chronic diseases, is a challenge to today's family doctor. In a predominantly white (Caucasian) population with the age/sex structure of the United Kingdom, 1·01% of the population will have diabetes. Of those over the age of 65, however, 3·5% will have diabetes and more than 50% of all diabetic individuals will be over the age of 65 years. With an ageing population this problem with numbers is likely to become an important factor for consideration in the provision of health care.[1] In an average practice list of 2250 patients there are likely to be 22 cases of diabetes known to the doctor and another 22 as yet undiagnosed.[2]

The Southall Diabetes Survey[3] highlighted a fourfold greater prevalence of diabetes mellitus among Asian immigrants to the United Kingdom. This is predominantly non-insulin dependent diabetes and tends to occur at a younger age than in the indigenous population.

45

There are additional problems in managing such patients and they mainly relate to difficulties in achieving understanding. In addition to problems with verbal communication, the patient must be considered in the context of such factors as religion, status within the family, and status within the community, as all these can influence the way in which the person reacts to illness and to professional advice on its management. Professionals should, when dealing with patients, be willing to adopt their modes of practice and to take account of these factors sensitively. Diabetes in the Asian community deserves more attention than it has so far received.

Diabetes can occur at any stage of life but its prevalence goes up with age. As the average age of the population rises, the long term complications of diabetes are becoming more common.[4] A particular concern for general practitioners is that, compared with the rest of the population, people with diabetes have twice the risk of a stroke or myocardial infarction, five times the risk of developing gangrene, 17 times the risk of renal failure, and 25 times the risk of blindness.

In spite of these known risks for patients with diabetes, there is evidence[5] that many general practitioners are not looking after their diabetic patients as well as they should. *Balance*, the patients' newspaper published by the British Diabetic Association, often cites cases of patients knowing more about their condition than their general practitioners do.

The requirements imposed on patients in guiding them towards optimal control are justifiable only if it can be shown that achieving such control will let them live longer with fewer complications. The following information is therefore important.

A prospective study of 4000 patients between 1947 and 1978[6] showed that complications were worse in those with poor control: there was a higher incidence of complications such as retinopathy, neuropathy, and nephropathy. Good control has a clear inverse relationship with retinal disease.[7] Close control of diabetes can arrest the progress of early retinopathy: patients allowed a freer regimen undoubtedly deteriorated.[8] There was no significant retinopathy in people whose blood glucose levels were kept below 11 mmol/l,[9] and retinopathy is also unusual in patients whose glycosylated haemoglobin levels are kept below 10%. The severity and frequency of acute neuropathic attacks are decreased by better control.[10] Triglyceride levels in diabetic individuals are directly related to those of glycosylated haemoglobin,[11] which in turn depends on overall blood glucose levels over the preceding 6–10 weeks. Cataract, a significant complication of diabetes, is undoubtedly associated with poor blood glucose control.[9]

For many decades, physicians have worked on the principle that the better the control of diabetes mellitus, the less the risk of long term vascular complications. Although this seemed logical, the proof for such a relationship was at best circumstantial until the last decade. More definitive proof became available in the summer of 1993 when the results of the Diabetes Control and Complications Trial (DCCT) were reported in the *New England Journal of Medicine*.[12]

The number of people aged between 13 and 39 years with type I diabetes who took part in this 10 year study in 29 centres in the United States of America and Canada was 1441. Half of the patients received "conventional" insulin treatment and half received intensified insulin treatment, either by means of multiple injection regimens or by using an insulin pump for subcutaneous insulin administration; dosages were guided by frequent blood glucose monitoring. Patients were followed for a mean of 6·5 years, and the appearance and progression of complications were assessed regularly.

Two cohorts of patients were studied: a primary prevention cohort in which patients had no evidence of vascular complications and a secondary intervention cohort to determine whether intensive therapy slowed progression of complications already present. The results were so conclusive that the study was stopped a year early for ethical reasons.

In the primary prevention cohort, intensive therapy reduced the adjusted mean risk for development of retinopathy by 76% compared with conventional therapy. In the secondary intervention cohort, intensive therapy slowed the progression of retinopathy by 54% and reduced the development of proliferative or severe non-proliferative retinopathy by 47%. In the two cohorts together, intensive therapy was associated with a 39% reduction in microalbuminuria (predictive of the later development of overt nephropathy), 54% in overt macroalbuminuria, and 60% in clinical neuropathy.

It is very important to state that the level of glycaemic control required to achieve these results was somewhat above the accepted normal range for both mean blood glucose and glycosylated haemoglobin levels, suggesting that the achievement of these goals is a practical proposition. In the words of Professor Harry Keen, speaking on behalf of the British Diabetic Association:

> This is one of the most important studies ever done for people with diabetes. It clearly shows that improved management of the condition will protect against long term complications. It shows that really tight control has dramatic effects and also that any degree of improvement will provide some reduction of risk of complications.

The St Vincent Declaration[13]

Representatives of government health departments and patient organisations for all European countries met with diabetes experts under the aegis of the Regional Offices of the World Health Organization and the International Diabetes Federation in St Vincent, Italy on 10–12 October 1989. The following recommendations were agreed unanimously and the representatives urged that they should be presented in all countries throughout Europe for implementation:

- Diabetes mellitus is a major and growing European health problem, a problem at all ages and in all countries. It causes prolonged ill health and early death. It threatens at least 10 million European citizens.
- It is within the power of national governments and health departments to create conditions in which a major reduction in this heavy burden of disease and death can be achieved.
- Countries should give formal recognition to the diabetes problem and deploy resources for its solution. Plans for the prevention, identification, and treatment of diabetes, and particularly its complications (blindness, renal failure, gangrene and amputation, and coronary heart disease and stroke), should be formulated at local, national, and European regional levels.

Investment now will earn great dividends in terms of reduction of human misery and massive savings of human and material resources. General goals and five year targets can be achieved by the organised activities of the medical services: in active partnership with diabetic citizens, their families, friends, and workmates, and their organisations, and in the management of and education about their own diabetes; in the planning, provision, and quality audit of health care; in national, regional, and international organisations for disseminating information about health maintenance; in the promotion and application of research.

The following are the general goals for people, children, and adults with diabetes:

- Sustained improvement in health experience and a life approaching normal expectation in quality and length
- Prevention and cure of diabetes and of its complications by intensifying research effort.

The declaration set out some specific targets:

- Reduction in new blindness resulting from diabetes by one third or more
- Reduction in numbers of people entering end stage diabetic renal failure by at least one third.
- Reduction by one half of the rate of limb amputations for diabetic gangrene
- A cut in morbidity and mortality from coronary heart disease in diabetic patients by a vigorous programme of risk factor reduction
- Achievement of pregnancy outcome in the diabetic woman approximating that of the non-diabetic woman.

It is interesting to note that the St Vincent declaration preceded the publication of the DCCT study by some four years, although the publication of the study has gone a long way towards justifying the faith of those responsible for the St Vincent Declaration.

What are our therapeutic aims and standards?

Our aims can be summarised as follows:

- To search for diabetes
- To stay in touch with people who are known to have diabetes
- To control blood sugar within an agreed range
- To search for early signs of end organ damage
- To ensure appropriate actions.

Here we might consider the words of AB Kurtz:[14]

> The goals of therapy are set by doctors but have to be achieved by patients.

The standards presented here follow from the aims set out above.

The search for diabetes and early and accurate diagnosis—Diagnosis is not difficult when the patient presents with the classic symptoms of thirst, polyuria, and weight loss. Other signs may be tiredness, pruritus vulvae, balanitis, blurred vision, ulcerated legs and feet (features of neuropathy), intermittent claudication, and recurrent sepsis. If a patient presents with any of these conditions a urine test or blood sugar estimation is indicated.

A fasting blood glucose level of over 7·8 mmol/l is almost always indicative of diabetes, as is a random blood glucose level exceeding 11 mmol/l. Diabetes is unlikely if the fasting level is below 6 mmol/l and the random level below 8 mmol/l.

Where blood glucose levels lie between these figures a glucose tolerance test can be useful. It is not necessary to perform the test routinely on patients with symptoms of diabetes whose blood glucose measurements are above 8 mmol/l (fasting) or 11 mmol/l (random sample).

The following conditions should be observed when carrying out a glucose tolerance test:

- The patient should have had normal carbohydrate meals for three days before the test. If he or she has been ill or has taken prolonged bed rest during this time the test should be postponed.
- The test should be done in the morning after an overnight fast.
- The patient should not smoke on the day of the test.
- The blood glucose concentration is measured fasting, then the patient is given a drink of 75 g anhydrous glucose in 250–350 ml water, and the concentration is measured every hour for two hours. Some doctors measure only the fasting level and the level two hours after giving the glucose; others prefer three estimations—fasting, one, and two hours after the glucose.

Table 4.1 shows blood glucose values based on the criteria of the World Health Organization. More generous values can be allowed in elderly people, especially in women. There is no point in upsetting the life of an elderly person who is asymptomatic and free of complications based purely on the result of a glucose tolerance test. Younger patients should be given dietary advice, especially if they are overweight, and should be reviewed periodically. *Pregnant patients with elevated blood sugar levels should be referred to a clinic specialising in diabetic care.*

Staying in touch with known diabetic patients—Once patients have been diagnosed as diabetic their names must be entered on a

Table 4.1—Blood glucose values based on World Health Organization criteria

Glucose tolerance test	Glucose concentration (mmol/l)		
	Whole venous blood	Capillary whole blood	Venous plasma
For diabetes mellitus			
Fasting	7	7	8
2 h after 75 g glucose load	10	11	11
For impaired glucose tolerance			
Fasting	7	7	8
2 h after 75 g glucose load	7–10	8–11	8–11

Source: World Health Organization Expert Committee on Diabetes Mellitus, 2nd report. *WHO Tech Rep Ser* 1980;**646**.

register that is updated regularly. If a register is not kept patients will usually be remembered within about six months by the doctor or receptionist, or from a request for a repeat prescription or the patient making an appointment, but this is hardly the way to run an efficient practice.

The diabetes register makes it possible to recall patients regularly. The frequency of recall depends on: how well the patient is managing the disorder him- or herself; the degree of control achieved; and the presence of other conditions such as infection, neuropathic ulcers, or hypertension, which would demand more frequent attendance.

Controlling blood sugar levels—For all patients with diabetes (whether or not they require insulin) diet is an essential part of the treatment. Changing dietary habits is always difficult, and the best way to do it is to start from the patient's usual diet. Competent dieticians can give invaluable help, and it is to be hoped that in future they will work much more closely with primary care teams.

In planning a diet the following principles apply to all patients with diabetes:

● The diet should be individually tailored and regularly updated to allow for age, weight, work and hobbies, and ethnic preferences. For non-insulin dependent diabetic patients and diabetic patients of normal weight taking tablets, the diet should provide enough energy for the patient to carry on with his or her job and recreations while maintaining an ideal body weight.

51

- In overweight patients the aim should be to reduce the total calories and so achieve ideal body weight (easy to say but difficult to achieve because some people use energy more efficiently than others).
- Increasing consideration is being given to the total energy content of the diet of the patient with diabetes rather than its carbohydrate component alone. (One gram of carbohydrate gives 17 kJ/4 kcal, 1 g protein the same, 1 g fat 38 kJ/9 kcal and 1 g alcohol 29 kJ/7 kcal.)
- Although in the past carbohydrate was quite severely restricted, it has now been suggested that it should contribute 50–60% of the energy produced by a patient's diet.
- Most of the carbohydrate should be starches rather than sugars, because starches are absorbed more slowly.
- The diet should be high in fibre.
- Use of polyunsaturated fats rather than saturated (animal) fats may reduce cardiovascular risk and should be encouraged.

In the light of the above information, a healthy diet can be achieved best by decreasing its fat, sugar, and alcohol content, and increasing the proportion of high fibre carbohydrate so that it contributes over 50% of the total dietary energy—for example, by including dried peas, beans, and sweetcorn. Such foods also slow the absorption of carbohydrate after a meal.

Common sense should be applied to the occasional binge, especially with children, for whom there should be ways of judiciously incorporating treats into the diet—for example, a "mini" Mars bar before exercise, or a sweet after a high fibre meal. We are all human.

First we shall consider measures for patients who are not dependent on insulin. If the patient is *overweight*—that is, two or more times the ideal body weight—try diet alone for three months. Then review the diet and compliance. If control has been achieved and the fasting blood glucose level is above 8 mmol/l, add metformin, starting with 500 mg twice a day. (Always check blood urea and serum creatinine first and bear in mind that metformin should not be used in patients with renal impairment, or for heavy drinkers.) Check control by measuring fasting blood glucose at monthly intervals, always reviewing the diet. If control has not been achieved, increase the dose of metformin progressively up to a maximum of 850 mg three times a day. If a month on this dose does not achieve control you should seek specialist help.

Patients should test their urine regularly for glucose and record the results.

If the patient is of normal weight try diet alone and review after one month. If control has not been achieved, even through the patient complies with the diet, try adding a sulphonylurea drug. If during the month's trial weight loss continues and/or ketonuria develops, earlier review is imperative. Then review monthly; consider diet and compliance and, if these seem satisfactory, increase the sulphonylurea in steps to the maximum dose for that particular drug.

Patients should carry out regular urine tests for glucose and, if this is above 2%, also for ketones.

If, after a further three months on maximum dose, control has not been achieved add metformin. If after another three months there is still no control consider insulin injections.

At all the decision points outlined above it is wise to reassess diet and compliance, and consider the possibility of infection before changing treatment.

Now we shall consider patients who depend on insulin. The drug can be used in several ways, the three most common being the following:

- Two injections of a short and medium or long acting preparation together, morning and evening
- In elderly patients, a single injection of a long acting insulin
- A single evening dose of a long acting preparation supplemented the next day by several injections of a short acting one. This regimen is likely to become increasingly popular in view of the results of the DCCT trial.

In deciding whether it is necessary to adjust the dose of insulin blood glucose monitoring is not only more useful than urine testing in patients with insulin dependent diabetes mellitus but is often more acceptable. For patients on two doses of short and medium or long acting insulin together, if glucose registers too high at one of the following times the basic rules are:

- *Breakfast*—raise the evening medium or long acting dose (but also beware of nocturnal hypoglycaemia)
- *Lunch*—raise the morning short acting dose

- *Evening meal*—raise the morning medium or long acting dose
- *Bedtime snack*—raise the evening short acting dose.

For patients on a single long acting injection, unmixed, base the decision to adjust insulin mainly on the morning blood of urine glucose level.

With the recent trend towards stricter control of blood glucose levels minor hypoglycaemia is inevitably more common. Doctors and nurses looking after diabetic patients should be sensitive to the fears of relatives that the patient may suffer a severe hypoglycaemic reaction. When a patient has an attack of hypoglycaemia the cause should always be sought and discussed with the patient.

The management of ketoacidosis is often a hospital task, but it is within the remit of the general practitioner to identify its cause and discuss this with the patient. The condition is almost always preventable.

Searching for early signs of end organ damage—Check the integrity of the skin. Look for ulceration or infection. Where necessary refer for chiropody. Check the peripheral pulses, dorsalis pedis, and posterior tibial. Examine the eyes for cataract and then, through a dilated pupil, for retinopathy. Once a year check for micro-albuminuria or frank albuminuria and monitor the serum creatinine. Check the integrity of the tendon reflexes in the lower limbs and for vibration sense at the ankle. Monitor the blood pressure regularly because the control of hypertension is particularly important in a diabetic patient. Control of blood pressure is second only to control of blood glucose in diabetics.

Ensuring appropriate action—Treat early complications vigorously; for example, treat skin infections with antibiotics and raised blood pressure with appropriate drugs. Make appropriate referrals. For example, if retinopathy is discovered refer the patient to an ophthalmologist; if hypertension cannot be effectively controlled refer the patient to a physician with a special interest in diabetes and hypertension.

Which aspects of performance need to be measured?

We need to know how many patients have had an annual review. We also need to know the proportion of diabetic patients who have had the following:

- Glycosylated haemoglobin measured at least twice yearly
- Cholesterol measured yearly or more often if necessary
- Creatinine measured yearly
- Periodic checks on injection techniques and blood glucose testing, as appropriate.

For each patient we should know the following:

- How often he or she has consulted us
- The number of episodes of hypoglycaemia that have occurred
- The number of times he or she has been admitted to hospital because of ketoacidosis or other diabetic complications
- How many days he or she has lost from work or school through diabetes or related conditions.

We should record the number of diabetic patients with complications affecting, for example, the eyes, feet, kidneys, or cardiovascular system.

What needs to change?

The first need is to review the present state of care in the practice for patients with diabetes, and to decide whether it can meet the aims set out above.

Does the practice have a protocol for the management of diabetic patients? If not, is it willing to develop one or to adopt one produced by another group such as the Royal College of General Practitioners?[15]

In the case of particular shortcomings the following five actions are recommended:

1 If the number of patients on the diabetic register is considerably smaller than would be expected from the age and sex distribution of the population, *check the diabetes register once more, using the repeat prescription system.*
2 If patients are not having eye checks, *review the resources available and consider referring them to an ophthalmic optician.*
3 If control of "diet alone" patients is inadequate, *review diet sheets and consider further help from a dietician.*
4 If data on blood pressure or chest pain are poor, *conduct partnership reviews and training of practice nurses.*
5 If hypoglycaemic attacks are too frequent, *review patient education and revise dosage schedules.*

Are all the practice's diabetic patients known and, if so, are their names entered on a register?

Are there facilities for estimating blood glucose, glycosylated haemoglobin, cholesterol, and creatinine?

Can a system be set up for patients to have an annual review? If not can an alternative strategy be devised?

What resources are available or required?

Time—If we are to care properly for patients with chronic conditions, such as diabetes, we have to find time and that time needs to be protected. Some practices have ensured this by setting up a specific diabetic clinic with defined hours. Time has to be protected for two reasons: first, it takes a long time to assess the needs of patients and their families and find how to meet them; second, professional workers such as nurses, dieticians, and chiropodists need time to meet and pool their skills for the benefit of the patient.

Space—In such a diabetic clinic workers clearly need a protected space of their own, both to carry out their work and to meet.

Records—Proper records are essential for any form of organised care. There should be a standardised record card on which information can be entered in a way that allows it to be easily compared with the findings of previous visits to the clinic (fig 4.1). There is much to be said for a system that allows information to be transmitted between primary and secondary care. The patient held diabetes record card of the Royal College of General Practitioners fulfils all these aims. An example of such a card is shown in the figure on pages 57–61.

People—The most important person at a diabetic clinic is the patient, who needs the support of skilled and compassionate carers. Ideally these should include a family doctor with a particular interest in the condition, a practice nurse who has developed skills in the care of diabetic patients, a dietician, and a chiropodist. These should in turn be supported by the practice manager and ancillary staff, who can ensure that the appointment system runs smoothly and can chase up defaulters.

Not all diabetic clinics in general practice will have the services of a dietician and chiropodist, but it should be possible to refer

THIS IS THE PERSONAL RECORD CARD OF:

Name.. D.O.B..................................... M/F

Address.. Tel. No. ....

....

GP.   Diabetic Liaison Sister   Consultant

Name........................... Name........................... Name...........................

Address......................... Address......................... Address.........................

....

Tel. No........................... Tel. No........................... Tel. No...........................

SIGNIFICANT EVENTS	DATE	NOTES

© THE ROYAL COLLEGE OF GENERAL PRACTITIONERS

Fig 4.1—Cooperation record card

patients quickly. Health districts developing a policy for patients with diabetes should make sure that these facilities are readily available.

Date of Diagnosis ....

PRESENTATION e.g.　Ketoacidosis
　　　　　　　　　　Routine Urine Test
　　　　　　　　　　Recurrent Sepsis

Criteria for Diagnosis

R.B.S.　　　　　　　　mmol/l　　　　　　(> II plasma glucose)

+ /or F.B.S.　　　　　　mmol/l　　　　　　(> 8 plasma glucose)

+ /or O.G.TT
　　75G 2 hour glucose　mmol/l　　　　　　(> II)

FIRST EXAMINATION

Height ....　Weight ....　Ideal Body Weight ....

URINE　　　Glucose　　Ketones　　Protein

B.P.　　　　Lying　　　　　　　　Standing

EYES　　　　　　　　　　　　R　　　　　L

　V.A.
　Fundi　　　　　　　　O　　╳　　　╳　　O

FEET

PULSES	R	L	REFLEXES	R	L	SENSATION	R	L
P. Tib			Knee					
D. Pedis			Ankle					

INITIAL MANAGEMENT PLAN

DIET　　　　　　　　　　　　　　　　OBJECTIVES

TABLETS

INSULIN

Fig 4.1—*contd.*

FOLLOW UP

Date	Diet	Insulin	Tabs	Loss Work School	Hypos	Inj-Sites	GHb	Notes

FIRST ANNUAL REVIEW   Date.................................

PROBLEMS: WELL BEING:

Smoking   Alcohol   Diet   Hypos

Insulin   Tablets   Photos

EYES   R   L   Date
  V.A.
  Fundi   O   ⋈   ⋈   O

PULSES	R	L	REFLEXES	R	L	SENSATION	R	L
P. Tib			Knee			Pin Prick		
D. Pedis.			Ankle			Vibration		

B.P.   Standing   Lying
GHb   Creatinine
Changes   Cholestrol
                                                Objectives

FOLLOW UP

Date	Diet	Insulin	Tabs	Loss Work School	Hypos	Inj-Sites	GHb	Notes

SECOND ANNUAL REVIEW   Date.................................

PROBLEMS: WELL BEING:

Smoking   Alcohol   Diet   Hypos

Insulin   Tablets   Photos

EYES   R   L   Date
  V.A.
  Fundi   O   ⋈   ⋈   O

PULSES	R	L	REFLEXES	R	L	SENSATION	R	L
P. Tib			Knee			Pin Prick		
D. Pedis.			Ankle			Vibration		

B.P.   Standing   Lying
GHb   Creatinine
Changes   Cholestrol
                                                Objectives

Fig 4.1—*contd.*

FOLLOW UP

Date	Diet	Insulin	Tabs	Loss Work School	Hypos	Inj-Sites	GHb	Notes

THIRD ANNUAL REVIEW   Date.................................

PROBLEMS: WELL BEING:

Smoking   Alcohol   Diet   Hypos

Insulin   Tablets   Photos

EYES   R   L   Date
V.A.
Fundi   O   ⬚   ⬚   O

PULSES	R	L	REFLEXES	R	L	SENSATION	R	L
P. Tib			Knee			Pin Prick		
D. Pedis.			Ankle			Vibration		

B.P.   Standing   Lying
GHb   Creatinine
Changes   Cholestrol
                                              Objectives

FOLLOW UP

Date	Diet	Insulin	Tabs	Loss Work School	Hypos	Inj-Sites	GHb	Notes

FOURTH ANNUAL REVIEW   Date.................................

PROBLEMS: WELL BEING:

Smoking   Alcohol   Diet   Hypos

Insulin   Tablets   Photos

EYES   R   L   Date
V.A.
Fundi   O   ⬚   ⬚   O

PULSES	R	L	REFLEXES	R	L	SENSATION	R	L
P. Tib			Knee			Pin Prick		
D. Pedis.			Ankle			Vibration		

B.P.   Standing   Lying
GHb   Creatinine
Changes   Cholestrol
                                              Objectives

Fig 4.1—*contd.*

FOLLOW UP

Date	Diet	Insulin	Tabs	Loss Work School	Hypos	Inj-Sites	GHb	Notes

FIFTH ANNUAL REVIEW   Date................................

PROBLEMS: WELL BEING:

Smoking   Alcohol   Diet   Hypos

Insulin   Tablets   Photos

EYES   R   L   Date
  V.A.
  Fundi   O   X   X   O

PULSES	R	L	REFLEXES	R	L	SENSATION	R	L
P. Tib			Knee			Pin Prick		
D. Pedis.			Ankle			Vibration		

B.P.   Standing   Lying
GHb   Creatinine
Changes   Cholestrol
          Objectives

BRITISH DIABETIC ASSOCIATION

National Address...

....

Local Address ....

....

Patients Notes...

....

....

....

Fig 4.1—*contd.*

Patient and family education—The principles outlined below should be borne in mind:

- Before starting any educational programme define its aims and objectives
- Checklists are useful, but remember that each patient is unique
- Tailor the programme to the patient and not the patient to the programme
- Do not offer too much too quickly: start with a basic package
- Teaching sessions should not be prolonged; offer the most important items first
- Make full use of literature and teaching aids that can be taken away by the patient and studied at home
- Information from all members of the primary care team should be consistent
- Continue educating the patient.

Equipment—Professionals running a diabetic clinic need the following:

- A register
- A call and recall system
- Record cards
- Booklets for patients to record results of blood glucose monitoring or urine testing
- A good weighing machine
- Snellen test charts for measuring visual acuity
- A good ophthalmoscope, blood pressure machines, and stethoscope
- A tendon hammer
- A tuning fork
- Tropicamide 2% eye drops to dilate the pupil
- Blood glucose testing strips.

Specialised diabetic clinics—Some patients—those with complications such as hypertension, renal failure, and ischaemic limbs—will need the expertise of a specialist clinic. Specialists should be consulted in a spirit of collaboration and not be allowed to take over the patient's case. Many people believe that children and pregnant women with diabetes should be looked after mainly by specialist clinics. My own view is that, if they are, they should not lose touch with their general practitioner clinic.

Optometrists—These have skills which can be applied to eye screening for patients with diabetes. Diabetic patients are entitled to free eye examinations if referred by their general practitioner. Optometrists will always agree to examine diabetic patients at least once a year and a regular arrangement can be made for them to do so.

Clinical pathology—Good relationships should be set up with local departments and with the chemical pathologist, and arrangements agreed for all patients to have their glycosylated haemoglobin regularly measured and the quality of their blood glucose monitoring assessed. The clinical pathologist's advice on the interpretation of results can be invaluable.

What is our performance now?

Has a suitable protocol been identified or developed in the practice?

Once the decision has been made to run a clinic, the first task is to identify patients. An up to date disease register makes this simple. If there is none you will have to rely on memory and repeat prescriptions as already described; this method may miss those patients whose condition is controlled by diet alone and who rarely test their urine. Has responsibility for maintaining and updating the register been given to a specific person?

Have the diabetic patients in the practice been identified and registered? The register should contain 1–2% of the practice population.

Is there a call and recall system for all the patients?

Are those patients who are not dependent on insulin seen at least twice a year and those who are dependent on insulin every four months?

Are the practice ophthalmoscopes suitable for screening? If necessary has training in ophthalmoscopy been arranged for those principals who will run the clinic? Alternatively, have arrangements been made for eye screening by a specialist clinic or local optometrist?

Are the following checks carried out on patients?:

1 At each visit the patient should be asked about problems that have arisen since the last visit; then the results of blood and urine tests should be studied, and the diet and dosage of tablets

or insulin reviewed. The patient should be weighed and his or her feet inspected. Blood should be tested for random blood sugar and, if 6–10 weeks have elapsed since the last visit, it should also be tested for glycosylated haemoglobin, especially in patients who depend on insulin. Urine should be checked for albumin. Injection sites should be inspected.

2 Periodic checks may be made on the patient's technique in drawing up and injecting insulin and in testing urine and blood glucose.

3 Once a year there should be a check of visual acuity and, after dilating the pupil, an inspection of the optic fundus. Also creatinine should be checked each year, and so should blood pressure, taken with the patient both lying and standing.

4 Regular checks on diet by a dietician are highly desirable.

Adequate documentation is essential, both so that findings can be compared with earlier ones and to make the recall system work properly. The card of the Royal College of General Practitioners has already been mentioned.

There is much to be said for making the patient's next appointment before he or she leaves the clinic.

Ideally, each primary care team should put one of its members in charge of the organisation and smooth running of the clinic.

Practice based diabetic clinics, which deal with relatively small numbers of patients and can offer continuing and personal care, should be highly acceptable to patients and satisfying for the primary care team.

Asthma

Asthma affects about 10% of the adult population and 15% of children, and there is some evidence that its prevalence is rising. Many have attempted to define asthma. The definition of Scadding[16] achieves the greatest clarity:

> Asthma is a disease characterised by wide variations over short periods of time in resistance to flow in intrapulmonary airways.

Before this century it was believed that asthma was never fatal, but it is now recognised that mortality from asthma can be as high as three in 100 000 patients each year in some countries. The highest rate is in New Zealand, followed, in decreasing order, by

Australia, the United Kingdom, other European countries, and North America.

Recent mortality figures from several countries have shown high rates in those aged between five and 34, a range in which diagnosis is likely to be accurate. In the United Kingdom today about 200 people die annually from asthma and, significantly, more than one third of these are under 55 years old.

Deaths from asthma are not decreasing—in fact they may be increasing. We still do not fully understand the condition, but I do not think that this is sufficient reason to explain why people die as a result of asthma. Better understanding will no doubt come, but meanwhile we have to find ways to stop deaths from asthma.

In 1979 a confidential inquiry conducted by the British Thoracic Society suggested that 86% of deaths from asthma could have been prevented.[17] In 1986 a working party of the Royal College of General Practitioners came to a similar conclusion, with a figure of 80–90%.

An overall impression from studies of asthma mortality is that patients die because their disease is not properly controlled; there is much evidence that asthma is underdiagnosed and misdiagnosed, and that its severity is not always properly appreciated.

We have many potent means of controlling asthma. It would be well to consider the words of VM Drury:[18]

> Our deficiencies are in the main due not to ignorance of new knowledge but to failure to apply existing knowledge.

Nothing, perhaps, exemplifies this better than asthma care. The safe and effective drugs we have had since 1970 for the treatment and prevention of asthma should have improved care for patients with the disorder. We still, however, have a legacy of underdiagnosis, undertreatment, and lack of patient education and proper follow up.

What are our therapeutic aims and standards?

Our aims are as follows:

- To search for and identify all patients with asthma.
- To keep in touch with all patients known to have asthma.
- To control the asthmatic state so that life is disrupted as little as possible by absence from work or school. Life should be as full and free as possible.

65

- To ensure that patients understand their condition and the aims of treatment.
- To let patients know what to do when their condition is deteriorating.

Standards follow from these aims.

Finding patients with asthma—In diagnosis the main requirement is for the clinician to be aware and suspicious.

Apart from asthma there are few disorders that cause recurrent wheezing in children. Diagnosis should not be difficult if a good clinical history is elicited, even if the child is not seen during an acute episode. The possibility of an inhaled foreign body should, however, always be considered in a toddler who presents with a first episode of wheezing. A child who wheezes in association with upper respiratory viral infections has asthma, not recurrent bronchitis. Sometimes in children the wheeze is not normally audible, but if, on auscultation of the chest, widespread wheezes are present asthma is probable, as it is when there is a recurrent dry cough at night.

Exercise can often bring on symptoms in children.

In adults the common presenting complaints are of tightness in the chest, wheeze, and dyspnoea. Diurnal variation in airflow is a most important diagnostic feature of asthma, symptoms invariably being worse on waking in the morning and being accompanied by a feeling of tightness in the chest. Nocturnal episodes of wheezing are another important feature, but in some patients it is nocturnal coughing not nocturnal wheezing that is the only symptom of asthma.

Bronchial hyperactivity—an essential feature of asthma—may be reflected in the patient's symptoms. Wheezing and chest tightness may be reported as a response to cold air or smoke. Some may report wheezing in response to drugs, specifically salicylates and non-steroidal anti-inflammatory drugs. Exercise can induce asthma attacks in adults, but less commonly than in children.

There is no need for elaborate investigations to make a diagnosis of asthma. By far the most important procedure is to measure ventilatory function, the most usual way being measurement of peak flow. Isolated or occasional measurements usually do not truly reflect the patient's condition. Far more valuable is a series of measurements obtained by a patient who has been trained to take his or her own measurements of peak expiratory flow rate.

Once patients with asthma have been identified they must be entered on a register which is regularly updated. This will at first consist only of newly diagnosed patients. The names of other patients with asthma need to be found from the memories of doctors, nurses, and receptionists, by monitoring repeat prescriptions, and checking surgery appointment lists.

Keeping in touch with patients who are known to have asthma—The register allows a planned recall system to be developed. No asthmatic patient should leave a consultation without being clearly told when he or she will be seen next. The frequency with which a patient's condition should be reviewed depends on its severity and how well it is controlled, how often acute episodes recur, and the confidence of the patient in managing the disorder.

Controlling the asthmatic state—Adequate control is shown by: a series of peak flow readings at or as near normal as possible; the least possible disruption of life, with no absence from work or school, no disturbed nights, no need to cancel social engagements; and, in children, adequate growth rate.

Understanding asthma and coping with deterioration—Patients should know that when their symptoms become worse they should immediately start monitoring their peak expiratory flow rate. If this falls to 70% of the predicted value they should increase the use of their steroid inhaler to four times a day (the usual dosage is twice daily). If peak flow rate falls to 50% of the predicted value they should start a course of oral steroids, 40 mg/day for adults and 20 mg/day for children, and contact their general practitioner.

Which aspects of performance need to be measured?
- The number of patients in the practice who are diagnosed as having asthma and are on the asthma register.
- The frequency with which patients are reviewed. Are intervals too long or too short? For example, two hospital admissions between review appointments would indicate that the interval is far too long.

- Some assessment of each patient's understanding of his or her disorder—that is, whether the patient can recognise deterioration objectively and knows the appropriate action.
- Simple measurements such as the number of nights disturbed by asthma attacks, the number of days lost from work or school, the number of courses of oral steroid therapy over a given period (say one year), the number of hospital admissions, and how many patients have developed virtually resistant airway obstruction—that is, their peak flow rate cannot be improved by intensive bronchodilator or steroid therapy.
- Level of smoking and what advice has been given.
- The patient's occupation.

What needs to change?

Primary care teams should take a much more proactive attitude to the diagnosis and management of asthma than the usual approach, which is essentially one of crisis intervention. Asthma should be seen as a notable example of a common disease which, although potentially serious, can and should be managed by the general practitioner.[19]

A primary care team adopting a proactive approach must either develop a protocol for the management of patients with asthma or adopt one produced by another group—for example, that of the Royal College of General Practitioners.[20]

Asthma is thought to affect about 10% of the population. The size of the practice's asthma register should be checked to see if it is reasonably near that percentage of the total register. If not the practice needs to step up the search for patients with asthma, reviewing the clinical criteria for diagnosis mentioned earlier and checking repeat prescription lists.

If patients do not follow your advice on treatment it is probably because they do not understand its aims. If examination of your own notes shows a lack of data on peak flow rates this probably calls for a partnership review and perhaps for the practice nurse to instruct the patient further.

A patient whose asthma is often exacerbated should have a review of how well he or she understands the disorder and complies with treatment. If you can find no fault with his or her understanding or compliance consider obtaining the opinion of a specialist.

The most important resources are an interested and knowledgeable general practitioner and practice nurse who can communicate clearly. Many patients with asthma can have their condition monitored during ordinary surgery consultations, but there may be advantages to setting up a specific asthma clinic.

Such a clinic can be run by a suitably trained nurse: the Asthma Training Society conducts courses for practice nurses. Little equipment is needed, the most important being plenty of mini-peak flowmeters and different types of inhalers for demonstration purposes. Peak flowmeters are now available on prescription and all but the mildest of asthmatic patients should have one (see *BMJ*, 28 February 1994). Serial peak flow readings can alert the patient to deterioration and thereby trigger effective action.

There is much to be said for giving patients simple instruction cards giving such information as:

My predicted peak flow reading is . . . If this drops to 75%—that is, . . .—increase the steroid inhaler to four times daily. If it falls to 50%—that is, . . .—take eight 5 mg prednisolone tablets a day, and contact the doctor. The practice number to ring for an appointment is . . . The practice number to ring for a home visit is . . .

Patient and family education—The principles outlined in the section on diabetes apply equally here.

What is our performance now?

- Has the practice either developed a suitable protocol or identified one that it can adopt?
- Has the practice compiled a register of its asthmatic patients and do the numbers on the register tally with the likely prevalence of asthma in the practice population? Has someone taken clear responsibility for maintaining and updating the register?
- Does the practice have enough peak flowmeters and demonstration equipment?
- Are all the patients on the register covered by a planned call and recall system with a frequency suitable for the severity of each person's condition?
- Is each patient's case reviewed periodically and is his or her understanding of the disorder assessed?
- Are the simple measurements referred to on page 68 recorded?

At this stage the practice should move towards auditing outcome. Deaths from asthma are likely to be rare in any one practice but overall their number is still too high, despite the effective measures that are now available to manage asthma. There should be a detailed review of any deaths; if necessary colleagues in secondary care should be involved.

It is in patients' best interests for their asthma to be managed by their general practitioner because he or she can offer better continuity of care than an outpatient clinic can, where they may be condemned to seeing a succession of junior hospital doctors with little experience or understanding of the long term care of their condition.

1 Gatling W, Houston AC, Hill RD. The prevalence of diabetes mellitus in a typical English community. *J R Coll Physicians Lond* 1985;**19**:248.

2 Tasker PRW. Is diabetes a disease for general practice? *Practical Diabetes* 1984;**1**(1):21–4.

3 Mather HM, Keen H. The Southall Diabetes Survey: Prevalence of known diabetes in Asians and Europeans. *BMJ* 1985;**290**:151–3.

4 Sönksen PH, Judd SL, Lowy C. Home monitoring of blood-glucose. Method for improving diabetic control. *Lancet* 1978;**i**:729–32.

5 Wilks JM. Diabetes—a disease for general practice. *J R Coll Gen Pract* 1973;**23**:46–54; Day LJ, Humphreys H, Alban-Davies H. Problems of comprehensive shared diabetic control. *BMJ* 1987;**294**:1590–2.

6 Joplin GF *et al. Proceedings of the 7th Conference of the International Diabetic Federation. International Conference 231.* Amsterdam: Elsevier, 1970. (Excerpta Medica International Congress Series No 276.)

7 Pirart J. Why don't we teach and treat diabetic patients better? *Diabetes Care* 1978;**1**:139–40.

8 Kohner EM *et al. Treatment of diabetic retinopathy.* Washington: US Public Health Service publication 1890, 1969.

9 Jarrett RJ, Keene H. Hyperglycaemia and diabetes mellitus. *Lancet* 1876;**ii**:1009–12.

10 Ward JD, Barnes CG, Fisher DJ, *et al.* Improvement in nerve conduction following nerve treatment in newly diagnosed diabetics. *Lancet* 1971;**i**:428–30.

11 Peterson CM *et al.* Correlation of serum triglyceride levels and haemoglobin A1C concentrations in diabetes mellitus. *Diabetes* 1977; **26**:507–9.

12 Diabetes Control and Complications Trial. The effect of intensive treatment of diabetes on the development and progression of long term complications in insulin dependent diabetes mellitus. *N Engl J Med* 1993;**329**:977–86.

13 Euro-Diab Care. *Diabetes Care and Research in Europe: The St Vincent Declaration Action Programme.* World Health Organization, 1992.

14 Quoted in Waine C. *Why not care for your diabetic patients?* London: Royal College of General Practitioners, 1988:2.

15 Waine C *et al. Diabetes: a protocol.* London: Royal College of General Practitioners, 1985.

16 Scadding JG. Definition and clinical categories of asthma. In: Clark TJH, Godfrey S, eds, *Asthma*, 2nd edn. London: Chapman & Hall Medical, 1983.

17 British Thoracic Association. Death from asthma in two regions of England. *BMJ* 1982;**285**:1251–5.

18 Drury VWM. Audit in general practice. *J R Coll Physicians Lond* 1981; **15**:259–61.

19 Anonymous. Asthma—a challenge for general practice [Editorial]. *J R Coll Gen Pract* 1981;**31**:331.

20 Waine C *et al. Protocol for the care of patients suffering from asthma.* London: Royal College of General Practitioners, 1986.

5 Acute conditions

KAY RICHMOND

Acute presentations make up a large part of the workload in primary health care during surgery consultations, home visits, and out of hours calls. The nature, place, and frequency of presentation of such conditions will, in large part, determine the method of audit used. Other variables to be considered are the age and sex of the patients presenting, their disposal—that is, advice, prescription, or referral—and the likely course of the disease. The effects on the practice workload and the usual methods of coping will also need to be examined.

The conditions I shall discuss have been selected to enable examination of different aspects of primary health care and of the interface with the hospital and community health sector. Time scales and contents of the audits will vary with such factors as those mentioned above.

Upper respiratory tract infection

In 1991–2 the incidence of upper respiratory tract infection (ICD 9 codes 034, 460, 462, 463, 465, 475) was 2185 per 10 000 person years at risk.[1] This resulted in 2525 doctor consultations by 1921 patients. This represents a considerable workload for the practice. Are all these contacts between doctor and patient necessary or desirable for a self limiting illness? If not why not?

Dr Kay Richmond is a Principal Medical Officer in the Welsh office. She has written this chapter in a private capacity and the views expressed are her own.

Can, or should, we attempt to change this pattern? Could the time and other resources used be better spent elsewhere?

Therapeutic and organisational considerations

The incidence of rheumatic fever and acute glomerular nephritis was falling before the advent of antibiotics.[2] In 1991–2 the incidence of acute and chronic rheumatic heart disease, Sydenham's chorea, and acute and chronic glomerular nephritis (ICD 9 codes 390–398 and 580–583) was 0·3 per 10 000 person years at risk.[1] It is unlikely that antibiotics have contributed much to this decline. We know that about 40% of upper respiratory tract infections are caused by bacteria;[3] the remainder result from viruses. In 1991–2 follicular tonsillitis and quinsy (ICD 9 codes 463 and 475) made up 21·5%, and streptococcal sore throat and scarlatina (ICD 9 code 034) 0·4% of the incidence of such infections.[1] Thus the course of the disease and its outcome are unlikely to be affected by the use of antibiotics in 60–70% of cases. There is evidence that antibiotics do not influence the reattendance rate[4] and that social and psychological factors significantly affect their use.[5] Thus we cannot hope to influence the course or outcome of a large proportion of these illnesses by an excessive use of antibiotics. In addition we teach patients that minor illnesses need a consultation and thus diminish their confidence to manage such conditions themselves, helping to make them dependent on the doctor and unnecessarily increasing the workload of the practice.

Is there any way in which we can adjust these imbalances? An agreed policy on the use of antibiotics—for example, in patients who are toxic or have quinsy—should aim to reduce their use where possible while advice to patients on how to manage upper respiratory tract infections themselves—for example, through the use of paracetamol or aspirin for three days before deciding whether a consultation is necessary—will increase their self confidence and help them to learn how to use the health care services most effectively. This should lead to fewer consultations, enabling the team to free time for other work—child health surveillance, for instance. Such a strategy applied to upper respiratory tract infections and other minor illnesses has been shown to work. In my own single handed practice over the period 1982–7 consultations fell from 5·3 to 4·6 per patient per year, in spite of immunisation and immunisation uptake levels in excess of 90%, a cervical screening level of 86% (plus 6% who had had a

73

hysterectomy) in women aged 35–64, and a blood pressure screening level of 95% in adults aged 20–64.[6]

The audit

To determine the current levels of performance in the practice it will be necessary to agree an audit protocol. What will need to be measured and recorded? Who will be responsible for keeping the records? Who will do the analysis and present the results?

As a result of the frequency and pattern of occurrence of upper respiratory tract infections it will probably be enough to carry out an audit over only one or two winter months. As 80% of consultations take place in the surgery it may be easier from an organisational point of view to audit only patients seen there. It may, however, be that the most ill patients are seen at home. Thus to exclude home visits may remove from the audit those most likely to receive and/or need antibiotics. It would therefore be preferable to include all patients presenting with upper respiratory tract infections over the agreed period.

If the partners agree to put to one side the notes of all patients seen with such infections the collection of data can be undertaken by the practice manager or nurse or one of the partners. An agreed proforma would considerably ease this task.

The data that need to be collected include the following:

- Where was the patient seen and when (surgery, home visit, out of hours)?
- The presence or absence of exudate
- The presence or absence of lymphadenopathy
- The presence or absence of pyrexia
- Was the patient toxic?
- Was a prescription issued?
- If so was it for an antibiotic, antipyretic, or antihistamine, and which one?
- Was self help advice given; if so what?
- How many times was the patient seen for this episode?
- Total practice consulting rate—in surgery, at home, out of hours.

When such data are analysed one can assess the feasibility of reducing prescriptions and increasing self help advice, thus influencing the demand for intervention in future. It may also be possible for the practice nurse to have a role in managing minor illness.

The lessons learnt

Once the current performance of the primary health care team and patients has been analysed, the use of published evidence should make it possible to consider whether changes are needed. If changes are agreed how can they best be implemented? When the new system has been in operation for a time the audit should be repeated to find out what effect the changes have had. It would be best to carry out this task one year later. As the second audit would be done at the same time of year as the first, seasonal effects would be removed, although not the effects of an "epidemic" year. The consulting rates for the year ending with the first audit and the subsequent 12 months could be compared to see if there had been any overall effect on the practice workload and if this was beneficial. Prescribing analyses and cost (PACT) data could be used to find the effect on prescribing behaviour. Finally, a value judgment based on the objective evidence will have to be made on the cost/benefit profile of the exercise and the practice's future policy for dealing with upper respiratory tract infection.

Hip, distal radial, and vertebral fractures

This subject heading is intended to show how acute problems can be audited to shed light on the way the team has looked at preventive medicine and the way in which an acute occurrence can act as the signpost to long term problems so that strategies designed to mitigate the effects can be planned.

The incidence of fractures of the neck of the femur, of the distal radius, and of vertebrae has been shown to increase significantly in people over the age of 65, particularly women.[7] Hip fractures are two to three times more common in women than men aged over 35 whereas Colles' fractures are six to eight times more common.[7 8] In 1985, 71% of hip fractures were in women aged over 65, and 3·4% of all hospital admissions for this group were in this category.[7] Of those able to walk before the fracture at least half are unable to do so independently afterwards.[7] Effective rehabilitation could significantly reduce this level of handicap.[9 10] Overall, about 30% of women are at risk of developing an osteoporotic fracture before 90 years of age.[8] Nevertheless, a survey of general practitioners in 1987 revealed that 20% stated that they had never seen a case of osteoporosis.[7] Clearly something is amiss.

75

Therapeutic and organisational considerations

The screening methods available for osteoporosis are, at present, unsuitable for mass screening programmes. Measurements of bone mass do not differentiate reliably between those who will sustain fractures and those who will not.[7] Thus it is possible to predict the proportion of the population that will develop osteoporosis but not the risk of fracture to the individual. Strategies are therefore needed to reduce the incidence of osteoporosis in the entire population.

The best known method of decreasing the likelihood of osteoporosis in women is the prescription of hormone replacement therapy after the menopause. The effects on the incidence of breast cancer and cardiovascular incidents are not, however, yet fully understood and there is much controversy over the use of the therapy. As many as 50% of postmenopausal women may refuse it because it would mean the return to cyclical blood loss. The evidence for screening for osteoporosis has been thoroughly reviewed in an *Effective Health Care Bulletin*, published in January 1992, in which the lack of evidence for the use of hormone replacement therapy in preventing fractures in elderly women was highlighted.[11]

Factors other than hormonal ones are known to contribute to osteoporosis. These include slim body build, immobility, low calcium intake, smoking, and high alcohol intake. Strategies such as calcium supplementation are unproven.[12 13] Many of these factors overlap with other areas of concern in primary health care—for example, hypertension, life style, and dietary habits.

A review of osteoporosis published by the Office of Health Economics[7] suggests that the presence of two or more known risk factors in women who have passed the menopause should indicate the use of hormonal replacement therapy. In the review it was estimated that if hormone replacement therapy had been used for the 25% of women most at risk from osteoporosis in 1985 there could have been a 50% reduction in the incidence of hip fractures.

Thus an effective health education and prevention strategy in primary health care may lead to a decrease in the numbers of women sustaining these fractures.

The audit

The loss of bone density is thought to begin after the age of 30,[7] increasing rapidly after the menopause. Fractures are often not presented in the first instance to the general practitioner but are seen initially in the accident departments of hospitals. Therefore to audit this group of diagnoses it will be necessary to institute a system capable of extracting the notes of all female patients aged over 45 who sustain fractures. The practice will usually be notified of these cases by the hospital. If all hospital letters are seen by the doctors in the practice before filing this may simplify the exercise, otherwise the ancillary staff will need to be fully and carefully briefed.

The incidence of fractures that occur because of osteoporosis is too low for a population approach in all but the largest practices, but a case by case analysis could yield useful lessons in the first instance. Over time, patterns of behaviour will become clearer. In 1991–2 the combined annual incidence of these three fractures (ICD 9 codes 820, 813, and 805–806) was 352 per 10 000 person years at risk for women aged 75 or more, 52 for women aged 65–74, and 21 for women aged 45–64.[1] For a practice of 10 000 patients with 4·2% of its population being women in the 75 + year age group a total of approximately 15 such fractures could be expected over a period of 12 months. With 4·5% of the population aged 65–74 two fractures could be expected and with 10·5% of the population aged 45–64 two fractures could be expected. This gives an expected total of 19 fractures within a year.

The following factors concerning these patients will need to be noted both before and after the fractures occur:

- Age at the menopause (early menopause associated with increased risk of osteoporosis)
- Parity (increased risk if nulliparous)
- Family history (increased risk if mother had history suggestive of postmenopausal osteoporosis)
- Body weight (thin people at greater risk)
- Low calcium and/or fluoride intake (increased risk of osteoporosis)
- High protein intake (increased risk of osteoporosis)
- Smoking, heavy alcohol intake, immobility, steroid therapy (increased risk of osteoporosis)
- Poor vision, mobility, coordination (increased risk of falling).

The presence or absence of any of these factors will need to be carefully assessed to minimise the likelihood of future falls and to halt or decrease the rate of loss of bone mass.

The lessons learnt

The comprehensiveness of the team's health education and promotion strategies, health screening, and the use of the practice nurse and the health visitor may well need careful examination after such an audit. Also the need to involve social service departments will have to be considered. The future care of patients sustaining such fractures will need to be directed towards lessening the effects of the acute episode and the prevention of future falls, fractures, and other disabilities.

Infectious diseases

This audit is intended to show how examining the occurrence of infectious diseases can lead to an assessment of the effectiveness of an immunisation campaign.

During the measles epidemic of 1986 I was puzzled because neighbouring practices were seeing many more cases than I appeared to be seeing. A review of my notifications book for the relevant period revealed five cases, all in children aged 6–10 years. Further investigation of these children and of the cohort who should have received measles immunisation over the preceding few years revealed that the cases had all occurred in children who had not been immunised. These included two sisters aged six and seven years whose mother had always failed to bring the children for immunisation and whom I had failed to "catch" opportunistically, and three older children whose immunisation status had never been adequately assessed. The uptake of immunisation in the younger age group was 100%. Thus the pattern of measles notification was adequately explained and the advantages of a high immunisation uptake were highlighted. A serious failure to assess adequately the immunisation status of children new to the practice was also revealed and corrective steps were taken.

A study of a measles outbreak in an infant school[14] showed attack rates in immunised and unimmunised children of 0·9% and 52·8% respectively. Hastings *et al*,[15] in a study of a measles epidemic, showed that each child contracting measles was ill for an average of 10·8 days and that the general practitioner spent 26 minutes providing care.

Complications have been reported in one in 15 notified cases, with encephalitis having an incidence of one in 5000 cases, a mortality rate of about 15%, and 20–40% of survivors have residual neurological sequelae.[16] Poorly nourished and chronically ill children are more likely to have complications. Following the introduction of notification of measles in 1940, the annual notifications varied between 160 000 and 800 000, with the peaks occurring in two year cycles. Immunisation was introduced in 1968 and by the mid-1970s notifications had fallen to 50 000–180 000. A similar effect was seen on deaths from measles, with a drop from 1000 in 1940 to 90 in 1968 and an annual average of 13 in the period 1970–88. MMR vaccine was introduced in October 1988 with only 9985 notifications in 1991, with no deaths in 1990 or 1991.

A similar approach could be adopted for influenza, except that it is not a notifiable disease and care needs to be taken in any audit that a definition of the diagnosis is agreed and understood by all participants. However, the pattern of a 'flu epidemic brings it to one's attention rather more quickly than is the case for measles; there is also the advance warning afforded by the World Health Organization, the Public Health Laboratory Service, the Royal College of General Practitioners' spotter practices, and the spotter schemes in Wales and Oxford. A review of all the influenza cases seen over a whole winter could serve to assess the adequacy of application of the programme of immunisation advocated by the Joint Committee on Vaccination and Immunisation in its memorandum.[15] This committee is made up of a panel of experts, representatives of the Royal College of General Practitioners and the General Medical Services Committee, and observers from the armed forces and the four United Kingdom health departments.

The audit

Once the cases to be reviewed have been selected from the consultation lists for the period of the epidemic the notes will need to be sifted for the following factors:

- Did the patient belong to one of the groups for whom immunisation is recommended by the Joint Committee on Vaccination and Immunisation?
- Was the vaccine given?
- If so how long before the diagnosis was made?
- If not why not?

The answers to the last two questions may then lead on to organisational matters such as the following:

- Was the immunisation programme completed early enough in the year (for 'flu) or was the relevant cohort approached systematically (for measles)?
- If not why not?
- If the vaccine was not administered was this because the patient refused it or because he or she was not offered it or because he or she does not belong to a group for whom immunisation is recommended by the Joint Committee on Vaccination and Immunisation?

The lessons learnt

The answers to the above questions may raise such issues as the practice's knowledge of, and application of, the recommendations of the Joint Committee on Vaccination and Immunisation. Although many reasons are traditionally offered for failure to meet immunisation targets, the Peckham report[17] found that the main obstacles to a child's being immunised were the misconceptions among general practitioners about contraindications. This finding has also been reported by Pugh and Hawker,[18] Morgan *et al*,[19] and Carter and Jones.[20] Surveys of practices to ascertain the prevalence of contraindications have found very few for measles.[21 22] Concerted efforts to increase the uptake have produced rates as high as 97%.[23] Those practices with a team approach had better uptake rates than those where the general practitioner had sole responsibility.[17] In 1989 Liston *et al*[22] reviewed the performance of their programme and the use of a checklist by the practice nurse; only one contraindication (to pertussis) was found in 155 cases and the checklist allowed the smooth operation of the clinic run by nurses.

It would appear that where the practice is well organised and the Joint Committee on Vaccination and Immunisation recommendations are known and comprehensively applied, the uptake of immunisation programmes can reach the recommended WHO targets. This would significantly reduce mortality and morbidity levels for the diseases covered and reduced the workload of infectious diseases for the primary health care team. Another perspective is offered by monitoring infectious diseases, particularly in epidemic years, as a means of assessing the effectiveness of the practice's immunisation programmes.

Abdominal pain

Abdominal pain is a frequent presentation in primary health care. An audit by Edwards *et al*[24] showed that 89% were managed entirely in the practice, 15% were investigated by the practice, 11% were referred to hospital, whereas only 2% were true surgical emergencies.

Abdominal pain requires careful history taking, examination, and investigation, with referral to hospital as appropriate. The chain of events presents a number of areas for audit that will lead to examination of the role of the patient, the practice team, and the hospital service. Grace and Armstrong[25] found that agreement on the reason for referral between patients and general practitioners was only 49·3%, between consultants and general practitioners 48·8%, between consultants and patients 47·8%, and among all three parties 33·3%. Clearly there is much room for improvement in commmunication between all concerned.

Therapeutic and organisational considerations

The causes of abdominal pain are legion, extending from acute appendicitis to cholecystitis, renal colic, urinary tract infection, ectopic pregnancy, strangulated hernia, and many others. As well as diagnostic pitfalls there may be problems of delay in the patient seeking help, problems in contacting the doctor, overbooked and rigidly organised appointment systems, unhelpful reception staff, inadequate history taking and examination, inadequate investigation, and inappropriate treatment or referral. Edwards *et al*[24] found that the median figure for days of pain before consultation was two. There may be undue delay in obtaining the results of investigations or in finding a hospital bed, or long outpatient waiting lists and delayed or inadequate hospital replies. Mageean[26] found that just over half the patients discharged from hospital had seen their general practitioner before he or she had received any information, and that the content of communications was variable with important subjects often omitted; no communication was received for 11% of discharged patients. All facets of the process require careful examination.

The audit

As a result of the frequency of presentation of abdominal pain a prolonged audit period will not be needed. Three months will probably be enough. The notes of all cases occurring within the period will need to be identified by the doctors. If a proforma has been designed and agreed for the audit the practice nurse or manager can then obtain the information required. The following points will need to be included in the proforma:

- Time from the start of the illness to consulting the doctor
- Reason(s) for any delay(s)
- Investigations undertaken and their results
- Time between requesting or doing investigations and receiving the results
- Presumptive diagnosis
- Confirmed diagnosis
- Disposal method—prescription, advice, referral as inpatient or outpatient, request for domiciliary visit
- Reason for referral
- Ease or difficulty of referral
- Result of referral
- Time from referral to receipt of reply
- If admitted time from discharge from hospital to receipt of report
- Outcome of episode.

The lessons learnt

Review of this audit will cover many areas. In cases where the patient has delayed seeking advice the reasons will need to be explored. These could range from "I didn't want to bother you doctor" through difficulties in reaching the surgery, either by transport or telephone, overbooked appointment systems with no room for emergencies, to unhelpful receptionists. Organisational hurdles will have to be examined and ways of removing them explored. The practice leaflet may need to be rewritten so that instructions for contacting the surgery in emergencies are clear and concise. Appointment schedules may need to be changed to free time for possible emergencies—for example, leaving a number of appointments unbooked until the previous surgery or having a combination of appointments and "join the queue" arrangements. Receptionists who are too protective of their doctors may need to have their energies redirected with explicit instructions given on how to deal with urgent requests. Perhaps the attitude of the doctor needs adjustment: it may be that the receptionist is "piggy in the middle" between an irascible employer and a desperate patient.

The investigations undertaken, if any, will depend on the provisional diagnosis. For example, where there was doubt of a urinary cause was a urinalysis undertaken? If not why not? Were Labstix and/or a microscope available? What was the result of the investigation? Were appropriate actions taken as a result? If there was time to request hospital investigation what was the time between the request being made and the test being done? How long did it take for the results to reach you? Were the results helpful? Were the tests requested or done appropriate?

The presumptive diagnosis will need to be checked against the definitive one for accuracy. If there was disagreement what was the reason for it? Was the difference within reasonable limits? If not what lessons can be learnt?

If advice and/or prescriptions were given were they appropriate? Did they achieve the desired result? Might there have been a better way of proceeding? Did the treatment have any side effects?

In the case of hospital referrals the ease or difficulty in obtaining help will need to be known. If there was undue delay or difficulty should this be pursued with the relevant authorities?

The outcome of all referrals will need to be known. If the patient was admittd was the care satisfactory? Was a definitive diagnosis made? How long was the patient kept in? How promptly were you notified of discharge? What were the discharge arrangements? Was the discharge appropriate (for example, adequate care being available at home) and was the district nurse involved? If so was the level of care appropriate or adequate? In the case of elderly and disabled people it may have been appropriate to involve the social services department and seek an appropriate assessment of need under the continuing care guidance arrangements. After an inpatient admission or an outpatient referral a letter summarising the hospital's activities and the opinion of the consultant should be received. How long did this letter take to arrive? Were its contents comprehensive and relevant? Any areas of concern about the hospital's performance will need to be pursued with the consultant or management as appropriate.

At the end of the exercise we should be able to judge the outcome for the patient, the practice team, and the hospital and community health sector. Collation of all the facets discussed should be undertaken at the end of the audit and underlying patterns discerned. There is little point in undertaking such a thorough review unless the shortcomings and deficiencies revealed are rectified and a repeat audit done after an appropriate interval to ensure that the lessons learnt have been applied and all concerned have benefited.

Urinary tract infection

Doctors in primary health care are frequently presented with symptoms of urinary tract infection. In 1991–2 cystitis (ICD 9 code 595) occurred at an incidence rate of 120 per 10 000 person years at risk. Females were involved 16 more times than males, with the number of cases increasing at the 16–24 age band and continuing at a steady rate thereafter for women, whilst it rose slightly for men from this age group throughout adult life, such that the male:female ratios were 1:58 for 16–24 years, 1:29 for 25–44 years, 1:12 for 45–64 years, 1:8 for 65–74 years, 1:6 for 75–84 years, and to 1:3 for 85 years and over.

Therapeutic and organisational considerations

The most common presenting symptoms are dysuria and frequency, 50% of cases being associated with bacterial urinary tract infection.[27 28] Most of these infections are caused by *Escherichia coli*, and trimethoprim is probably the antibiotic of choice.[27] In half of these *E. coli* infections spontaneous cure can be expected within 72 hours.[27] Before writing a prescription one has to decide which cases are likely to be bacterial in origin.

The patient's discomfort is usually severe enough for there to be considerable pressure for an immediate diagnosis and treatment. Labstix and side room microscopy can be helpful.[27] Alternatively, the diagnostic methods described by O'Dowd *et al*[29] or Dobbs and Fleming[30] may be used. If a mid-stream urine specimen is taken it should be sent to the laboratory immediately or stored at 4°C until despatch is possible. Once a decision to issue an antibiotic has been taken the length of course will need to be considered and may vary between one and seven days.[27] However, 5–10% of infected patients will remain bacteriuric. Whether or not a prescription is issued appropriate advice on follow up and management of possible future episodes should be given.[28]

The audit

The collection of data will need to be made over a six month period and should cover the following points:

- Duration of symptoms before presentation
- Presence or absence of dysuria, frequency, nocturia, and incontinence
- Presence or absence of proteinuria and haematuria
- If a microscope is available the numbers of cocci and white blood cells in each high power field should be recorded
- Whether a pre-treatment urine specimen has been sent to the laboratory
- Result received from laboratory on pre-treatment specimen
- Advice given (verbal or written)
- Prescription given (which drug, dosage, duration)
- Follow up arranged
- Follow up attended
- Follow up urine specimen sent to the laboratory
- Result received from laboratory on follow up specimen
- Appropriateness of prescription
- Outcome.

The lessons learnt

Once again delays in presentation need to be considered. Can these delays be ascribed to the patients or to the practice? What can be done to minimise them in future?

The correlation of symptoms, diagnosis, management, and outcome should be examined. Were appropriate investigations carried out? Were the collection, transport, and examination of specimens satisfactory? If the results of hospital investigations were not received by the time of the patient's follow up visit, the reasons for this will need to be explored and negotiations with the appropriate people should be initiated to improve the service.

The Public Health Laboratory Service and other microbiology laboratories keep records of the results of all tests submitted. It would be useful to have regular updates of the results, particularly the organisms grown and their antibiotic sensitivities. If these updates are not already being provided it may be worth investigating the possibilities for the future; for example, it may be possible for a quarterly or annual update of the numbers and proportions of all specimens sent by general practitioners (urine samples may account for 40% of bacteriological specimens and samples submitted by general practitioners 10% of the overall workload)[29] together with a summary of the results to be circulated by the FHSA.

If advice on self help and prevention were not given why not? Appropriate patient literature may be obtained and handed to the patient during the consultation and displayed in the waiting room.

Accurate, timely, and caring management of urinary tract infection needs to be ensured to minimise the risk of recurrence and long term complications.

Acute diarrhoea

Most cases of acute diarrhoea seen in British general practice are caused by viruses.[31] In 1972 in England and Wales 297 children aged less than one year died of acute diarrhoeal disease—more than any other EC country except for Italy.[32] By 1992 the numbers of deaths from intestinal infection for this age group had fallen to eight.[33] The incidence of severe dehydration and hypernatraemia have been greatly reduced, probably because of the introduction of low solute milks and oral rehydration therapy. In contrast there has recently been an increase in the notification of food poisoning—13 124 cases in England and Wales in 1985, 20 363 in 1987, and 63 346 in 1992.[34 35]

Therapeutic and organisational considerations

In 1991–2 the combined incidence of intestinal disease of proven and presumed infective origin (ICD 9 codes 001–009) was 420 per 10 000 person years at risk, giving rise to 417 doctor consultations with 409 patients.

In 1979–80 and 1982–83 Kumar and Little[36] carried out two surveys of children admitted to hospital with gastroenteritis. The use of drugs dropped from 50% to 16% between the two surveys, and of those admitted 83% received oral rehydration in the first survey and 94% in the second. The children treated with drugs before admission needed to stay in hospital for longer. Another hospital survey in 1987–88[37] showed inappropriate treatment with drugs in 17% of cases and that 18% were not following the recommended guidelines for feeding during acute gastroenteritis. During hospital admission 88% were treated with standard oral rehydration solutions. A diagnosis of the postenteritis syndrome was made in 11% of children but all resolved satisfactorily within four months on a diet free of cows' milk and lactose.[38]

Diarrhoea may be prolonged in a small percentage of patients. It may result from the following factors:

- Postenteritis syndrome
- Salmonellae or shigellae: treatment with antibiotics is rarely needed and should be given only after expert advice
- *Campylobacter* sp.: treatment with erythromycin may be necessary
- *Giardia lamblia* or cryptosporidiosis: it may be necessary to use metronidazole
- Other causes: for example, typhoid fever if the patient has recently been abroad.

Any case suspected of being contracted from food or water will need to be notified to the Consultants in Communicable Disease Control so that the source of infection and contacts can be traced and measures taken to limit the spread of the infection. This is of particular importance with the current increase in food borne infections thought to result from inadequate storage and handling. These infections may also be attributed to food being stored for too long in fridges and freezers, to inadequate hygiene, and to failures in food preparation, such as food being cooked for too short a time.

Most cases of acute diarrhoea are seen and managed successfully in general practice, but you will need to know if the management has been appropriate.

The audit

The audit will need to take place over a period of from three to six months. As a result of the various ways in which patients may come to the notice of the health care team the notes of all patients with a relevant diagnosis (diarrhoea and vomiting, gastroenteritis, dysentery, etc) seen in surgery and at home by the doctor or nurse will need to be kept to one side for completion of the agreed proforma. In addition the post will need to be sifted to spot patients coming to light through hospital letters, from occupational health services, and the Consultants in Communicable Disease Control.

The data requiring collection should include the following:

- Place of presentation
- By whom seen

- Symptoms and signs
- Laboratory specimens and the results
- Advice given
- Treatment given, if any
- Consultants in Communicable Disease Control notified—yes/no
- Removed from work if a food handler—for example, cook, waitress, children's nanny?
- Hospital referral. Why, where, type?
- Outcome.

The lessons learnt

Analysis of the above data should enable you to answer such questions as these:

- Is our consultation rate for this problem high, average, or low? Are there any explanations?
- Was the patient seen by the appropriate person—nurse, doctor or hospital?
- Was there delay in presentation—if so why?
- Were appropriate specimens taken?
- Was appropriate advice given?
- Was appropriate treatment given, if any?
- Was hospital referral appropriate; what was the management there; was a timely and relevant letter received?
- Were the Consultants in Communicable Disease Control notified? Degree of liaison and outcome
- Were the process and outcome the best that could have been achieved? If not why not?

The particular points to be noted should include the appropriate use of staff, the appropriate use of oral rehydration therapy, the inappropriate use of antidiarrhoeals, antiemetics, or antibiotics, and appropriate or inappropriate referral to hospital and/or notification of the Consultants in Communicable Disease Control.

A repeat audit during the same months one year later will reveal if proper advice on oral rehydration therapy has, as well as being better for the patients, enabled greater patient autonomy and self confidence in handling minor illness with more appropriate recourse to the primary health care team where the course of the illness has been atypical or protracted, thus helping to make use of the team's resources more effectively and efficiently.

Summary

I have tried to show how the audit of acute conditions can be the route to wide and far reaching examinations of subjects rather than of the index conditions in isolation. The wider areas I have attempted to cover are appropriate prescribing, factors affecting workload, screening, acute conditions leading to chronic ones, health promotion and education, appropriate laboratory tests, appropriate hospital referrals, adequate communication between the primary health care team and the hospital and community sector, immunisation performance, and the interface with public health medicine. The types of audit covered should help you to examine the structure, process, and outcome of primary health care in your practice so that you may gain increased health and autonomy for your patients and greater job satisfaction for yourselves.

1 Royal College of General Practitioners, Office of Population Censuses and Surveys, Department of Health and Social Security. *Morbidity statistics from general practice: fourth national study 1991–1992.* Series MB5. No 3. London: HMSO, 1993.

2 Irvine DA. The general practitioner and upper respiratory tract infection in childhood. *Family Practice* 1986;3(2):126–31.

3 Marcovitch H. Sore throats. *Arch Dis Child* 1990;65:249–50.

4 Howie JGR, Hutchinson KR. Antibiotics and respiratory illness in general practice: prescribing policy and workload. *BMJ* 1978;ii:1342.

5 Howie JGR. Clinical judgement and antibiotic use in general practice. *BMJ* 1976;ii:1061–4.

6 Richmond JK. *The feasibility and cost of a screening and treatment programme for hypertension in general practice.* Part II project for the Faculty of Community Medicine. (In libraries of the Faculty of Public Health Medicine and the Royal College of General Practitioners.)

7 Griffin J. *Osteoporosis and the risk of fracture.* (Current Health Problems No 94.) London: Office of Health Economics, 1990.

8 Cooper C. Osteoporosis—an epidemiological perspective: a review. *J R Soc Med* 1989;82:753–7.

9 Kennie DC, *et al.* Effectiveness of geriatric rehabilitative care after fracture of the proximal femur in elderly women: a randomised controlled trial. *BMJ* 1988;297:1083–6.

10 Currie CT. Hip fracture in the elderly: beyond the metalwork. *BMJ* 1989;298:473–4.

11 *Effective health care: Screening for osteoporosis to prevent fractures. January 1992.* No 1. OIS University of Leeds, 1992.

12 Kanis JK, Passmore R. Calcium supplementation of the diet—I. *BMJ* 1989;298:137–40.

13 Kanis JK, Passmore R. Calcium supplementation of the diet—II. *BMJ* 1989;**298**:205–8.

14 Kimmance KJ. A measles outbreak associated with an infants' school. *Health Trends* 1989;**21**:40–1.

15 Hastings A, *et al*. Measles: Who pays the cost? *BMJ* 1987;**294**:1527–8.

16 Joint Committee on Vaccination and Immunisation. *Immunisation against infectious disease*. London: HMSO, 1992.

17 Peckham C, Bedford H, Senturia Y, *et al*. *The Peckham report. National immunisation study: factors influencing immunisation uptake in childhood*. Horsham: Action Research for the Crippled Child, 1989.

18 Pugh EJ, Hawker R. Measles immunisation: professional knowledge and intention to vaccinate. *Community Medicine* 1986;**8**(4):340–7.

19 Morgan M, *et al*. Parent's attitudes to measles immunisation. *J R Coll Gen Pract* 1987;**37**:25–7.

20 Carter H, Jones IG. Measles immunisation: results of a local programme to increase vaccine uptake. *BMJ* 1985;**290**:1717–19.

21 Kemple T. Study of children not immunised for measles. *BMJ* 1985; **290**:1395–6.

22 Liston A, *et al*. Use of a contraindications checklist by practice nurses performing immunisation at a well child clinic. *J R Coll Gen Pract* 1989;**39**:59–61.

23 Anderson PMD. Measles immunisation: what can we achieve? *Update* 1987;**1**(9):408–12.

24 Edwards MW, *et al*. Audit of abdominal pain in general practice. *J R Coll Gen Pract* 1985;**35**:235–8.

25 Grace JF, Armstrong D. Reasons for referral to hospital: extent of agreement between the perceptions of patients, general practitioners and consultants. *Family Practice* 1986;**3**(3):141–7.

26 Mageean RJ. Study of "discharge communications" from hospital. *BMJ* 1986;**293**:1283–4.

27 Brumfitt W, Hamilton-Miller JMT. The appropriate use of diagnostic services: investigation of urinary infection in general practice: are we wasting facilities? *Health Trends* 1986;**18**:57–9.

28 Pill R, O'Dowd TC. Management of cystitis: the patient's viewpoint. *Family Practice* 1988;**5**(1):24–8.

29 O'Dowd TC, *et al*. Sideroom prediction of urinary tract infection in general practice. *The Practitioner* 1986;**230**:655–8.

30 Dobbs FF, Fleming DM. A simple scoring system for evaluating symptoms, history, and urine dipstick testing in the diagnosis of urinary tract infection. *J R Coll Gen Pract* 1987;**37**:100–4.

31 Nicholl A, Rudd P (eds). *Manual on infections and immunizations in children*. Oxford: Oxford University Press, 1989.

32 Anonymous. More about infant diarrhoea [Editorial]. *BMJ* 1977;**ii**: 1562.

33 Office of Population Censuses and Surveys. *1992 Mortality statistics*. Serial DH2 no. 19. London: HMSO, 1992.

34 Office of Population Censuses and Surveys. *Registrar General's annual returns, 1987*. London: HMSO, 1980.

35 Office of Population Censuses and Surveys. *1992 Communicable Disease Statistics.* OPCS Series MB2. London: HMSO, 1992.
36 Kumar GA, Little TM. Has treatment for gastroenteritis changed? *BMJ* 1985;**290**:1321–2.
37 Jenkins HR, Ansari BM. A hospital survey of gastroenteritis in South Wales. *Arch Dis Child* 1990;**65**:939–41.
38 Wharton BA, Pugh RE, Taitz LS, *et al.* Dietary management of gastroenteritis in Britain. *BMJ* 1988;**296**:450–2.

6 Clinically significant events

GRAHAM BUCKLEY

Introduction

Audit is a mean, pernickety kind of word which is inadequate for the imaginative, stimulating activity which it seeks to describe. European general practitioners have preferred the term "quality assurance," which has a more positive ring to it. This chapter considers clinically significant events and so focuses on the heart of general practice—the consultation.

The only requirement for this type of audit is positive motivation by the doctor. No specialist registers or sophisticated information systems are needed, only the wish to become involved because of the realisation that we can all improve our clinical skills.

The field is a wide one: all consultations between doctors and patients are of clinical significance to at least one of the participants; this chapter covers the whole of general practice. Concentrating on single events is a simple and practical method of selecting important aspects of practice for scrutiny. One type of audit examines the processes of care associated with clearly defined outcomes—for example, births, deaths, emergency admissions to hospital, and adverse drug reactions. Another fruitful approach is to select consultations at random.

Medical audit is usually taken to mean an exercise involving the collection of quantitative information about groups of patients or about patterns of intervention within a health care system. This has been the main thrust of medical audit over the past 10 years.[1] The objectivity of this approach is commendable, but the relevance of quantitative information is doubtful if not placed in the proper context; for example, to make any judgment about the number of referrals by general practitioners to gastroenterologists it is necessary to know morbidity patterns within the practice, the availability of open access contrast radiology and endoscopy, and whether general physicians in the locality also see patients with gastrointestinal problems.

Restricting audit to aspects of medicine that are easily quantifiable and measurable excludes large and important areas of clinical practice. The medical anecdote has rightly fallen into disrepute as a valid way of advancing an argument about the best way in which to manage clinical conditions. The special circumstances and idiosyncrasies that are present in an individual case may preclude any general inferences being drawn. Nevertheless, the audit of single cases and single consultations is important in identifying issues that can be pursued and tested in other settings and on other occasions. More than other types of medical audit the analysis of single cases and single events defines and refines questions rather than providing answers.

I start my examples of medical audit of clinically significant events with random case analysis because it is a simple technique that reaches the core of general practice. General practice is unique in medicine in having no fixed boundaries. Our clinical work is determined by what patients think is appropriate to present, reveal, or hide. Random case analysis samples the whole breadth of general practice and permits audit to be vigorous yet open ended and open minded. I began this introduction by bemoaning the connotations of the word "audit." We must take care to prevent the reality of medical audit from becoming censorious, negative, and dispiriting. Provided that it is carried out with honesty and sensitivity in cooperation with trusted colleagues, the audit of clinically significant events will be sustaining and invigorating and consequently likely to be integrated into general practice to the lasting benefit of both doctors and patients.

Random case analysis

This approach to the evaluation of clinical skills has become established as a major element in the training of general practitioners. At its simplest the method requires just a list of patients seen at a recent surgery session. At a tutorial between a trainee and trainer it is the custom for the trainer to select a case from the list at random and question the trainee about it. The trainer and the trainee may learn more from this activity if from time to time the procedure is reversed and the trainer is questioned about his or her management of cases.

In a group of trainees, in a Balint group, or in other small discussion groups the technique can be adapted so that each participant brings a list of patients or agrees to describe the patient seen at a previously specified time—for example, the third patient seen on a Tuesday morning.

This simple technique is a robust and powerful method of revealing the way in which doctors consult but it depends on how the individual doctors perceive the consultation.[2] This inevitably biases subsequent discussion and evaluation. Audio and video recordings of consultations are free from this kind of bias but do introduce possible intervention effects into the consultation itself. The mechanics, acceptability, and evaluation of video recording consultations have been extensively described and discussed because of the unrivalled possibilities the technique provides for evaluating and learning interviewing skills. Although well established as part of vocational training, random case analysis is not yet a normal part of continuing medical education for general practitioners. Balint groups pioneered the use of routine clinical material as the basis for learning about the way in which patients and doctors interact. These groups continue to prosper but involve only a small number of self selected general practitioners.

Many general practitioners still seem reluctant to expose their consultation behaviour to the scrutiny of those with whom they work. Part of the reluctance may relate to the paradox which lies at the heart of clinical medicine. As scientists doctors learn to be sceptical and critical about current conventional wisdom and to keep open minds about the efficacy of therapeutic interventions, but as clinicians they discover the benefits of giving patients confidence in their diagnostic pronouncements and treatment recommendations. Apparent clinical confidence becomes part of the armamentarium of general practitioners, who nevertheless remain aware that this confidence does not rest on a solid foundation and can easily be punctured by peer review. Introducing random case analysis into continuing medical education needs to be done with care and tact. If this is achieved the rewards in terms of job satisfaction and improved team work could be immense.

An important principle to be adopted in all forms of random case analysis is to look for positive features before negative ones. The doctor under scrutiny should be given the first opportunity to describe the consultation and note the good features before commenting on the weaker aspects. Similarly, the trainer or peer group when discussing the case should also first identify good points rather than areas of weakness. Specific criticisms should be offered only when a better approach can be suggested. This procedure may seem to be excessively protective of the sensibilities of experienced professionals, but it is all too easy to concentrate in a destructive way on one small, weak aspect of a consultation that is otherwise effective.

Whatever method of random case analysis is used the types of questions asked will be similar.

Has the clinical problem been clearly identified?—Why has the patient come? Why today? Why to this particular doctor? These related questions are the starting point for understanding the consultation and are implicit in the opening remarks made by the doctor to the patient. The opening comments by doctors and patients are crucial in determining the way in which consultations proceed, and are likely to reflect previous encounters. Byrne and Long[3] showed how doctors can become stereotyped in their opening remarks on consultations. This may not matter if the remarks are welcoming but otherwise neutral and permit patients to raise issues in the way they wish.

It is possible to discuss at length the possible reasons for a patient consulting a particular doctor on a particular day. The reasons may be purely pragmatic and relate to constraints within the practice organisation. Questioning along the lines outlined above, however, may alert the doctor concerned to aspects of the consultation that had not previously been considered. It may place the content of the consultation in the appropriate context and influence the way in which the doctor starts his or her consultations in future.

Have underlying or continuing problems been declared or explored?— In the currently fashionable jargon the doctor and the patient may each have an agenda for the consultation that is not explicit at the outset and not part of the presenting problem. General practitioners are familiar with consultations in which patients reveal major health

95

problems or worries just before they leave. During consultations patients are assessing doctors and may use a relatively trivial health problem to judge whether the doctor may be willing to respond to other health problems. Video and audio recordings of consultations are the only way in which any judgment can be made about a doctor's ability to pick up clues about underlying health problems. The recording may reveal moments when the doctor could have offered the patient the opportunity to present additional health problems.

Stott and Davis[4] provided a model for the consultation that has received widespread acceptance. In this model, in addition to the management of the presenting problem, consultations can also include the management of chronic problems, opportunistic screening, and health promotion. Not every consultation will include these aspects of the doctor's agenda but if the pattern that emerges from random case analysis is for a doctor to concentrate exclusively on the presenting problem of the patient this area of questioning will challenge him or her.

What are the expectations of the patient from the consultation?— Doctors tend to assume that they know what patients expect from consultations and consequently they fail to check them out—for example, more patients receive antibiotics for sore throats than expect them. An important element in the consultation therefore is to clarify the expectations of the patient. Audio and video recording may show ways in which this aspect of the consultation is successfully dealt with and illustrates the way in which this technique is a powerful educational tool for observers as well as the observed.

There has been recent interest in the concept of heath beliefs. Deeply embedded attitudes concerning health appear to influence the way in which people use health services. Patients who rarely if ever see their doctor appear to have a strong sense of their own well being and resilience; other patients may be basically pessimistic about their own health and bring transient symptoms and minor health problems to the doctor for consideration. Random case analysis may reveal whether the doctor can place the present consultation in the context of the health career and health beliefs of the patient.

Do we have adequate information about the clinical problem?—Other questions are subsumed under this question such as: What investigations are required? Has a sensible treatment plan been formulated and explained adequately to the patient? In these aspects of a consultation doctors will feel more secure and confident because they relate directly to the training they receive. Elsewhere in this book emphasis is given to the creation of standards of care and the criteria by which health care is judged. It is true that in many clinical conditions, such as diabetes, epilepsy, or hypertension, standards of care can be established. One of the goals of clinical medicine is to establish standards of care on the basis of evidence and research. Much of general practice remains uncertain. Patients present with symptoms, not with diseases, and, in the absence of certainty, treatment may have to be on the basis of probabilities about the possible causes of symptoms or even just at the level of symptom relief.

For example, conventional standards for the management of urinary tract infection could be: adult women complaining of dysuria and frequency should have a pre-treatment specimen of urine tested bacteriologically; treatment should be on the basis of the sensitivity of the identified pathogen; and a sample of urine taken after treatment should be tested to demonstrate eradication of the infection. In practice there are difficulties with these standards. Mid-stream specimens of urine are not infallible in diagnosing urinary tract infections. The delay between the onset of symptoms and the identification of the infecting organism may be intolerable for some women, who may request immediate treatment with antibiotics. The general practitioner may feel that the balance of benefit lies in complying with this request and selects an antibiotic on the basis of local patterns of infection. In a personal audit of my management of suspected urinary tract infection in adult women less than 10% of the patients handed in specimens after treatment. Women who no longer have symptoms of dysuria and frequency do not have a strong incentive to hand in a further urine specimen. Population surveys indicate that up to 5% of women have asymptomatic bacteriuria. Population surveys also indicate that most women with symptoms of dysuria and frequency initially seek advice from a pharmacist rather than a doctor and only if symptoms persist for more than two or three days do they seek the advice of a general practitioner.

Perhaps a more sensible set of criteria for the management of women complaining of dysuria and frequency in general practice is as follows:

- Is there anything about the case that alerts the doctor to potentially serious problems? Is this a recurrent problem? Could the patient be pregnant? Is there a family history of renal problems? Does the patient have other health problems that may make the possible urinary tract infection potentially more serious (for example, diabetes)?
- Are there identifiable precipitating factors affecting the condition (for example, relationship to sexual intercourse)?

An audit evaluates whether a search for these features was carried out by the doctor. Other criteria can be advocated. Some doctors consider that it is important to have objective evidence of infection before treatment. They would wish to have the microscope examination of urine as a criterion of good care.

The difficulty in creating criteria of good care extends to many of the common conditions seen in general practice—for example, sore throats, earache, and respiratory tract infections. Although absolute standards of care cannot be set because of deficiencies in our basic knowledge and in our diagnostic abilities, we are still obliged to develop clinical policies that are sensible, consistent, and coherent. It brings no credit to the profession or to a particular practice if the treatment offered for these conditions varies according to the day of the week or with the particular doctor consulted. Audit exposes uncertainty as well as measuring performance against established standards.

How did the doctor feel about the consultation?—It is important in the analysis of a consultation for the doctor under scrutiny to be given the opportunity to describe how he or she felt about the consultation as a whole. Dissecting the consultation into its component parts is useful but the overall impact of the consultation should not be neglected. Consultations which technically may be deficient may nevertheless be worth while because of the empathy, genuineness, warmth, and concern displayed by the doctor. This is not to minimise criticisms of technical aspects of the consultation, but a consultation may be technically competent and yet be deficient in these general qualities. A patient who leaves a consultation believing that the doctor has taken an interest in his or her problem and is genuinely concerned in seeking a solution will be likely to return and provide the doctor with further opportunities for helping. A cool, detached doctor may have only physical problems presented by the patient, who may choose not to reveal important psychosocial dimensions to his or her problem.

Random case analysis is an important technique in medical audit as it demonstrates that all aspects of medical care are available for scrutiny. It is a necessary counterbalance to the view that much of general practice is amenable to the implementation of protocols. Each consultation is rich in human potential. The spark of genuine communication between a patient and a doctor may be ignited over apparently banal medical problems. We must guard against crushing spontaneity, imagination, and creativity in consultations because of external requirements to document, categorise, and report on their content.

In the rest of this chapter I look at different types of clinically significant events. The selection is idiosyncratic and arbitrary and starts with an event that is unlikely to figure in medical textbooks.

Heart lift

There have been several papers that have sought to define "heart sink" patients—patients whose name on a surgery list evokes gloomy anticipation on the part of the doctor. In pursuing the theme that audit should be about positive aspects of general practice as well as negative ones we need to draw attention to consultations that have a positive outcome for the doctor. Descriptions of these patients can be an enjoyable lead into random case analysis.

There is also a serious aspect to this exercise. In general practice doctors are likely to see 30 or more people each day. There is the danger of consultations becoming routine for the doctor so that the problems of patients are dealt with at a superficial level only. Or there is the opposite danger that general practitioners become overwhelmed or "burnt out" by the emotional needs and demands of patients. The antidote to these dangers is the humour, excitement, surprise, and uplift which consultations also produce. These motivating and energising feelings will be reinforced by sharing them with colleagues.

In the next section we consider more conventional clinically significant events by examining life events.

Life events

Births—In a list of 2000 patients there are likely to be over 20 births each year. Fortunately major obstetric problems are now rare and quantitative audit will be unlikely to be rewarding. Recording the number of mothers who breast feed their infants is worth while as a measure of the effectiveness of health education in the antenatal period. Detailed questioning of some or all of the mothers will provide qualitative information that might identify strengths and weaknesses in the care provided by the practice. Mothers may be more forthcoming to the midwife or health visitor than to the doctor and communication between the different members of the team could establish criteria of care against which information from the patient could be matched; such communication also identifies areas of care that cause concern for members of the team—for example, smoking during pregnancy. Some ways of formulating the aims of antenatal care are given below:

- The mother understands the purpose of antenatal clinics in identifying risk factors for delivery and in assessing the progress of her pregnancy
- The mother knows what to expect at different stages of labour and what action to take
- The mother is aware of the benefits of breast feeding and of how she can be helped to initiate breast feeding
- The mother knows how to seek help and advice about herself and the baby in the puerperium.

These have been set out as a list of objectives for the mother's knowledge and understanding because these can be ascertained by interviews with the mother in the first month after delivery of the baby.

If the audit has been jointly planned by the different members of the primary care team it is more likely that information gathered will then be acted on by the team. An audit by one profession in isolation could be seen as threatening by the other professions involved.

Marriage—Marriage is not yet seen in this country as a reason for visiting the general practitioner. Although a happy event, marriage is accompanied by changes in lifestyle that may be stressful. Notification of a change of name through marriage is an opportunity for a general practitioner to suggest a consultation to discuss family planning, provide preconceptual advice for the couple, and check whether the young married woman is immune to rubella.

Death—Less than a third of people die in their own homes and not all of the people dying at home suffer from illnesses that involve terminal care. On the other hand, many of the patients who die in hospices or in hospitals will have been cared for by the primary care team during their final illness. Research studies have shown areas of weakness in the services provided by primary care to the terminally ill and their carers. These weaknesses relate to the way in which information is provided and the inadequacy of symptom relief, especially pain control. Sensitively handled analysis of the care provided for the terminally ill can be of benefit both to the surviving relatives and to the primary care team. Feelings of guilt and anger are normal components of grief and these feelings may be present in all who cared for the dying person. Enlisting the help of the bereaved person could be therapeutic for the individual as well as beneficial for the service. Aspects of care that the bereaved carer could be asked about include the following:

- Frequency of visits by the general practitioner, district nurse, specialist nurse
- Continuity of care
- Symptom control—pain, bowel function, mental distress
- Communication with the patient, with relatives, within the health care team, and with specialist colleagues
- Timing of referral to hospital.

Suicide—Death by suicide is by any reckoning a clinically significant event. Suicide leaves a legacy of distress in the family of the dead person and a sense of failure in the health workers involved. Acknowledging and sharing these feelings in a discussion within the primary health care team will help the doctors and nurses cope and equip them to help in turn the relatives of the dead person. An honest evaluation of the factors leading to the suicide is necessary. There may have been extensive support given to the patient extending over many years, or even more tragically the suicide may appear to have been a sudden impulsive action by someone apparently well. Medicine and doctors do not have a monopoly of relevant skills. The spiritual dimension to this event is obvious and the involvement of a minister with the family and with the practice team may be welcomed. Guilt and forgiveness seem a long way from resource management and audit, but general practice is a long way, thank goodness, from the retail trade.

Medical emergencies

Chest pain—Each general practitioner is likely to be called to one or two patients each year who are suffering from acute myocardial infarction. A similar number of people will be seen who are suffering severe acute chest pain but who do not have myocardial infarction. Acute chest pain is a potentially life threatening event and it is important for practitioners to be able to respond quickly and effectively when informed about a patient with severe chest pain. The precise arrangements for responding to such a call will depend on geographical and other factors, but the following checklist will help to establish whether the practice can respond appropriately:

- Practice switchboard not overloaded; incoming calls answered quickly
- Telephone receptionist aware of the need to be able to respond quickly to a patient with chest pain
- General practitioner available and able to respond immediately to the call; contact procedure understood by reception staff
- Appropriate equipment and drugs immediately accessible.

This form of audit can and should be carried out without having to wait for the next emergency. Most of the delay between the onset of symptoms of myocardial infarction and treatment is because of the patient. Delay in treatment has an adverse impact on the prognosis after myocardial infarction. The development of thrombolytic agents in readily injectable forms emphasises this point. Practices will need to decide whether to stock them, and whether to have portable oxygen sets and to carry electrocardiograph and defibrillator machines. The quality of the local ambulance service and the proximity of the coronary care unit will influence the decision of the practice.

In reviewing the management of a case of myocardial infarction the procedures carried out can be reviewed and any weaknesses identified. Another important function in reviewing the case, however, is to determine whether there were any avoidable risk factors for the heart attack. Had the patient's blood pressure been checked? Was his or her smoking status known? Had the weight been checked in the past three years? Was there a strong family history? Following successful initial treatment of a person having a myocardial infarction, what assessments were made to help the patient achieve a return to full function? In attempting to minimise the risk of further attacks, is the lipid status of the person known and has the possibility of familial hyperlipidaemia been ruled out?

Epileptic fits and febrile convulsions—General practitioners are likely to be contacted when a patient has a first seizure. Although epilepsy as a chronic problem is common in general practice, the number of people experiencing first epileptic seizures is only likely to be one or two a year for each general practitioner. A practice may also expect to see one or two febrile convulsions.

The response of the practice to patients who present with their first seizure is considered in this chapter. The management of epilepsy as a chronic problem would follow the guidelines set out in the chapter on chronic conditions, though it is not specifically mentioned there.

There are a number of areas of possible concern surrounding the management of a first seizure. These include: management of the seizure itself; accuracy of the diagnosis and identification of possible causes; the understanding of the patient and his or her carers about the seizure and its implications for work and leisure activities; and the compliance of patients with recommended treatment regimens.

Analysing the way in which an emergency call is received may reveal different problems at different times of the day. Having received the call the doctor needs to be able to respond quickly and have available the appropriate drugs. Reviewing the clinical management of a seizure is likely to lead to a discussion among the partners in a practice about the best drugs for use in this situation. Agreeing a clinical policy, even if this policy specifies a range of drugs from which the individual doctor can choose, is a useful step if it leads to ensuring that these drugs are immediately available to the duty doctor.

After successful management of the seizure a decision has to be made whether to refer a patient to hospital. A number of factors will influence this decision; for example, in the case of a child a prolonged seizure and the absence of focal signs of infection would favour immediate referral to hospital because of the possibility of meningitis. An adult suffering a first seizure on withdrawing from heavy alcohol intake might not require immediate referral.

Justifying the particular decision made in a particular case helps to make these criteria explicit and so develops a practice clinical policy. It is this aspect of case review that makes the audit of clinically significant events an educational process for the doctors involved. Other aspects of the early management of seizures that can be included in a practice policy include the types of investigations to be carried out and whether to offer prophylactic therapy to patients after a first seizure.

Another important element in management is to check the understanding of the patient and relatives of the problem and its implications. The possibility of repeated seizures means that driving, unsupervised swimming, and other potentially dangerous activities must stop. Coming to terms with these changes in lifestyle may be difficult for some people and medical audit includes an evaluation of the way in which patients and their relatives react. Conventionally, the review of individual cases tends to rely on the written case record and the memory of the doctor concerned. There may be opportunities for inviting the patient to join in the review of the case. Alternatively, the views of the patient or the parents of a child who has had a febrile convulsion may be presented by means of a video recorded interview.

New diagnosis of malignant disease

The diagnosis of malignant disease is undoubtedly a major clinical event. The commonest neoplasms in men are lung cancer and large bowel cancer. In women carcinoma of the cervix and breast cancer are the malignancies that we are most likely to see. Taking all cancers together a general practitioner is likely to see about three new cases each year.

The areas of potential concern surrounding the diagnosis of malignant disease include avoidable factors, delay in diagnosis, communication with patient and relatives and with other agencies involved in care, and responsibility for continuing care. Many of the avoidable factors and delay in diagnosis may lie in the domain of the patient, with cigarette smoking and denial of symptoms common factors in men and avoidance of cervical cytology screening in women. Nevertheless, the occurrence of cancer, particularly carcinoma of the cervix, will cause a practice to question whether its health promotion and screening programmes are sufficiently active.

Questions in each of the categories listed in the box will be helpful in evaluating all clinically significant events.

In the case of malignant disease it is worth questioning whether the treatment offered to a patient was discussed adequately, in particular whether different treatment options were discussed with him or her. How the information about the diagnosis of malignancies is conveyed

- Avoidable factors
- Delay in response
- Intervention
- Communication
- Rehabilitation

to the patient and to relatives merits inquiry. Surveys suggest that many patients are not given a clear description of the nature of the cancer and are left to speculate on the extent of their problem.

HIV disease

The diagnosis of HIV infection poses problems for patients that are similar to those of malignant disease, with the added problems of stigma and the effects on sexual relationships. The first case of HIV infection in a practice provides the opportunity for educating the whole of the practice team. This can be achieved while maintaining confidentiality at the level requested by the patient. Many patients infected with HIV have shown themselves willing to discuss with health professionals the way in which they became aware of their illness and the effect that it has on them.

HIV tests need to be carried out in a variety of circumstances. Applicants for life insurance and for visas for some countries are sometimes required to have the test done. Increasingly people who think that they may be at risk of infection because of high risk sexual activity, intravenous drug use, or accidental exposure through injuries are asking for the test. In all cases people need to be aware of the implications of a positive and of a negative test. A review of a particular case would seek to establish whether enough information had been given to the patient before the test was done. Whatever the result of the test the patient needs to understand the need to avoid high risk behaviour in the future. In behavioural terms therefore a test is irrelevant and an individual may prefer the uncertainty of not knowing his or her HIV status to the certainty of a positive test. The provisional results of treating infected people at an early stage in their disease with zidovudine, however, indicate that there may be a practical benefit in confirming the diagnosis of HIV infection.

Before carrying out a test for HIV a policy on the way in which information about tests is to be handled within the practice should be established. Doctors, medical secretaries, and nurses should all be aware of the way in which test results are received and recorded. After discussion the practice may agree not to share information about a patient's HIV status.

All staff should be aware of the ways in which HIV can be transmitted, in particular the fact that the virus cannot be spread through normal social contact. A practice meeting about HIV infection is an opportunity to tighten up on clinical activities involving invasive procedure and on the way in which equipment is sterilised.

Counselling after the test has been done cannot be completed in a single interview. Patients who are found to have the antibody for HIV will be stunned when they are first told, and their capacity to take in additional information will therefore be limited. A second consultation is essential, and efforts should be made to ensure that the patient has the support of friends or relatives as he or she adjusts to the information. The prognosis needs to be given in a realistic manner, but this does not mean being unduly pessimistic. Many people remain well for many years and there have been significant therapeutic advances. Monitoring the level of CD4 lymphocytes, along with other features, provides a good prognostic assessment. The value of continuing supervision should therefore be emphasised. Before the test, counselling about social behaviour should be reinforced for the HIV positive person. Whether other people should be informed requires careful consideration. Sexual partners do need to be told, but unless the occupation of the patient involves putting other people at risk—for example, if the patient is a surgeon—there is no overriding need to inform anyone else. The extent to which information about a patient's HIV status should be shared within the practice team needs to be discussed explicitly. In an emergency it may be to the advantage of the patient if the duty doctor is aware of the HIV status, otherwise the diagnosis of *Pneumocystis carinii* pneumonia may be missed or delayed.

The House of Commons Social Services Select Committee stated that the care of people with HIV infection is important in itself but will also act as a guide to the adequacy of our health care system as a whole. General practice should be a major contributor in the care of people with HIV infection and AIDS. To make this contribution we need to demonstrate our willingness to participate, to develop clinical expertise, and to learn how to link with the specialist services and voluntary agencies that are already providing much of the care for these patients.

Sudden onset disability

A stroke or a fall resulting in a fractured femur is an event that transforms the life of one of our patients. Strokes and fractured femurs are common clinically significant events, but because in most cases the early weeks of treatment are in hospital the crucial importance of primary health care for these patients is not sufficiently recognised. Surveys have revealed the sorry plight in which many disabled elderly people often find themselves after they are discharged from hospital. An audit of the rehabilitation of these patients will necessarily cover the whole range of community services. The particular contribution of home helps, physiotherapists, health visitors, occupational therapists, district nurses, and general practitioners will vary from individual to individual. Much effort often goes into the multidisciplinary assessment of these patients before they are discharged, but it is rare for a systematic review of them to take place one or two months after they have left hospital.

Discharge from hospital could act as the trigger for an audit exercise in which all elderly people in a practice who had been discharged from hospital in the previous six months could be reviewed in a systematic way. The checklist below shows the areas that the review might cover. Medical audit tends to focus on the performance of doctors and other health workers; it can also evaluate the availability of resources. The audit may reveal that the major deficiency in the care of disabled older people is in the lack of resources in the community. Medical audit then becomes a means for lobbying the health and social service authorities; for example, the physical needs of disabled people may be being cared for adequately but loneliness is found to be a feature common to all the patients reviewed. This could support the case for providing transport to day centres for elderly people.

The following checklist could be used for assessing elderly people:

- Mobility and balance, indoors and outdoors
- Self care and continence—bathing and toileting
- Social support—relatives, neighbours, home help
- Nutrition—meals, teeth

- Mental status—mood, memory
- Foot problems
- Vision
- Hearing
- Medications—compliance, non-prescribed
- Finance—benefits
- Housing—hazards
- Review arrangements—general practitioner, health visitor, district nurse, frequency.

Referrals to a hospital

The new contract for general practitioners requires practices to provide information on the use made of hospital facilities. For budget holding practices the cost as well as the number of hospital referrals will need to be calculated. The government is interested in this aspect of general practice because three quarters of health service expenditure relates to the hospital services. Surveys have repeatedly demonstrated that there is a wide variation in the number and in the pattern of referrals made by general practitioners. The variation is reduced but still considerable if practices rather than individual practitioners are used as the denominator in calculating referral rates. Variations between doctors are not associated with any identifiable factors such as age, qualifications, or experience. Other than as a fiscal exercise simple quantitative analysis of the use of hospital services is unlikely to illuminate the quality of practice. To learn from analysing referrals to hospital it is necessary to place the quantitative data in the appropriate context. The use of hospital based facilities for investigations in general practice is considered in the next section. This is done to show how simple audit projects can be undertaken while at the same time demonstrating how difficult it is to draw any inferences about quality of care from the data.

Investigations

The simplest quality control type of audit projects in general practice assess the way chronic illness is monitored. For the patient this is not a clinically significant event and is considered in the chapter on chronic diseases. Most other investigations are, however, of clinical significance to the patient. The investigation indicates that the patient and/or the doctor considers that it is important to test for a possible physical cause for the problem presented by the patient.

Haematology, biochemistry, simple contrast radiology, endoscopic examinations, and computed tomography are examples of diagnostic services that may be directly available to a general practitioner. In the United Kingdom these services are usually hospital based.

The request for a full blood count is a common event in general practice and can serve as a model for the audit or more elaborate investigations. The basic questions for an audit project in this area are as follows:

- Can criteria be agreed within the practice concerning the appropriate use of the haematology service in carrying out full blood counts?
- Can data be gathered on all requests for full blood counts from the practice?

After discussion partners may agree on criteria similar to the following:

- It will be possible to state a reason for requesting a full blood count (1) in the anticipation of a normal result and (2) in the anticipation of an abnormal result
- The test result, whether normal or abnormal, will have an impact on the subsequent clinical management of the patient
- Procedures for informing the doctors and patients of the test result will be reliable
- Partners will have similar ratios of abnormal to normal test results.

The practical procedure may be conducted along the following lines. The haematology department may be able to identify the source of samples for full blood counts by the practice and doctor. The laboratory is likely to provide only sample numbers, but new computer facilities may make possible the identification of individual patients. The laboratory may be able to state whether the total number of requests is similar to that from other practices of equivalent size. More precise comparisons of numbers of requests may be possible by agreement with other practices.

It is helpful if the practice keeps a register of all samples sent to hospital laboratories. This is useful for checking the date of despatch of samples and other data that may enable a missing result to be tracked down. From the register it will be possible to calculate the number of requests for full blood counts made by each doctor over a period of two months. This length of time is chosen because it is likely to identify about 30 requests by a particular doctor and within the short time period doctors may be able to recall details of the consultations not recorded in the patient's notes.

For each request for a full blood count the doctor is asked the following questions:

- Was the request made at the first or at a subsequent consultation for the presenting problem?
- Reason for the request?
- Was the test expected to be normal or abnormal?
- Did the result influence subsequent management of the patient?

Experience from previous studies indicates that it is likely that there will be considerable variation between doctors in any group practice in the number of requests made. Suppose that in a five doctor practice Doctor A arranged for 60 tests of which 16 were abnormal and Doctor D arranged for 15 tests of which eight were abnormal. In all the cases both doctors thought that the test results influenced their subsequent management of the patients.

In the absence of other information it would be easy to draw the erroneous conclusion from these data that Doctor A is profligate in his use of laboratory investigations and that Doctor D may be missing some cases of anaemia in the patients he sees. At a simple operational level there may be factors that contribute to the difference in pattern beween the two doctors. Doctor A may conduct most of the antenatal clinics in the practice and be required to send blood for full blood count as part of the overall local clinical policy on antenatal care; Doctor D may only consult in the afternoons when access to the haematology laboratory is difficult.

Nevertheless, these figures are likely to be the starting point for a discussion within the practice about the workload of different doctors, the case mix of patients seen by different doctors, and the threshold for investigation for different doctors. In the absence of quantitative data it is difficult for doctors to discuss how they respond to patients with ill defined symptoms such as feeling tired. Audit of this kind does not demonstrate that the doctors with high or low rates of investigation are right or wrong in their clinical practice. All doctors who participate in this type of clinical review are stimulated to question their own patterns of behaviour and are given the opportunity to learn from the ways in which other doctors manage common clinical conditions.

Clinical mistakes

In chapter 1 Marshall Marinker highlights the need for doctors to learn from their mistakes. Error in clinical medicine is inevitable. Our knowledge of disease, physiology, and human behaviour will always be less than perfect, as will our knowledge of our own strengths and weaknesses.

Each year a general practitioner is consulted between 4000 and 10 000 times and the average length of a consultation is less than 10 minutes. The range of problems brought to a general practitioner is wide. Consequently, in spite of high volume, the number of patients with a particular disease is small and it is difficult to maintain technical expertise in a specific area of practice. These characteristics of general practice mean that errors will be frequent and they should be regarded as normal. As yet, however, errors have not been regarded as an important resource for medical audit or continuing education.

Fortunately most errors in general practice are not dramatic or life threatening but this does not diminish their potential value in indicating ways in which clinical practice can be improved. Honest discussion of a perceived clinical mistake could not only prevent a recurrence of the error but also reveal systematic problems within a practice that require tackling.

Before giving examples of the ways in which clinical mistakes can be utilised in medical audit it may be helpful to explore the barriers to this type of audit. No one enjoys admitting to error. This innate reluctance is compounded in medicine by our early clinical training. Public humiliation on teaching ward rounds soon convinces the more sensitive medical student that the most important skill is not to avoid error itself but rather to avoid the exposure of error. This lesson may be reinforced when as a house officer the most pressing requirement is not to help patients but to keep consultants happy by providing them with cosmetic versions of the truth. This is an overstated description, but it is fair to say that there is no active encouragement in medical education to learn from the inevitable errors that occur.

There is a need to separate error from blame. Blame and the fear of litigation are a barrier to our learning from our mistakes. Anything that goes wrong in medicine is now seen as the basis for legal action.

This is damaging in the long run for patients and for doctors. Attempting to prove medical negligence is difficult, lengthy, and costly for patients. Fear of litigation may lead doctors to overinvestigate their patients and focus attention unduly on physical aspects of ill health.

For medical audit into clinical mistakes to prosper a climate has to be created in which uncomfortable episodes can be freely discussed. Such a climate can be most easily achieved in a peer group of doctors. This may be the partners in a practice or a small discussion group of colleagues from different practices.

The first example describes how one mistake was handled within a practice.

Drug allergy

At a practice meeting Dr Brown described a visit she had made to a Mrs Walmsley, who had developed a severe rash affecting the whole body. The patient was cross because she felt that the rash was similar to but worse than a previous drug reaction to a sulphonamide. Dr White had visited her three days before Dr Brown saw her and had prescribed co-trimoxazole for a urinary tract infection. The patient had assumed that the doctors knew that she was allergic to sulphonamides; only later did she realise that one of the ingredients of the prescribed antibiotic was a sulphonamide. Dr Brown and Dr White had already discussed the case before the meeting and had identified a number of points that they wished the partners to consider.

1 The original call had been made at 9 pm on Sunday evening. The symptoms had been present for two days but were increasingly severe and Mrs Walmsley complained of blood in the urine as well as frequency and dysuria. On the telephone Dr White ascertained that there had been no significant previous medical problem and did not pick up the medical records before visiting the patient. On his way to Mrs Walmsley's house he received a potentially more serious call via his pager. As he was already nearly outside Mrs Walmsley's house he decided to see her before visiting the next patient.
2 Dr White thought that he had asked Mrs Walmsley about possible allergies to antibiotics.
3 Reviewing Mrs Walmsley's notes did not reveal any information about previous drug reactions on her summary card but

continuation notes before 1980 had been removed by a previous doctor.

What would be the probable outcome of the practice meeting? The detailed discussions and possible changes in the arrangements for out of hours calls and in the data held in medical records can be left to the doctors concerned. The fact that the problem was discussed in a constructive and open fashion is of prime importance. Initially Dr Brown shared some of the patient's sense of outrage that this problem could have occurred. It would have been easy for the sake of superficial harmony within a practice for the episode to have been glossed over without resolving these feelings. The meeting allowed Dr White to understand the cumulative factors that contributed to the problem. As a result of the meeting not only Dr White but all the partners are likely to be more searching in future in eliciting possible drug allergies before prescribing.

What about the patient? After the practice meeting Dr White contacted Mrs Walmsley, who had now recovered both from the urinary tract infection and from the drug rash. She was invited to come and discuss her experience and at the consultation she was offered an apology and informed that the practice had discussed the problem and steps were being taken to avoid a recurrence. Mrs Walmsley was impressed by the serious way in which her problem had been taken up. On her part she would be certain to alert any future doctor about her drug allergy.

Wrong injection

A young principals' discussion group had been meeting each month for a year. As part of each meeting one doctor presented a recent clinical problem. On this occasion Dr Steven described her most recent immunisation clinic. By mistake she had omitted to give pertussis immunisation to a baby and had only given diphtheria and tetanus toxoids. Although the mistake was not of any immediate significance, Dr Steven was concerned that it had occurred and was in a dilemma about what she should do to rectify the mistake. Would informing the mother diminish her confidence in the practice? What would be the best way for the baby to catch up on pertussis immunisation?

The meeting, which had been in danger of sinking into torpor, suddenly became lively and animated. A consensus soon emerged about the practical steps to be taken. Most of the doctors felt that the mother should be informed straight away and offered a choice between an immediate pertussis immunisation for her child and a short wait until the next routine second immunisation, with a subsequent catching up for pertussis.

For Dr Steven the surprising aspect of the discussion was the interest shown by the other doctors in the precise arrangements for the immunisation clinic. Did she conduct the clinic alone? Who was responsible for recording the immunisations in the medical records and updating the practice and health board computer file on immunisations? How many children were seen at each session? From questions such as these it became clear that different practices organised clinics in very different ways. Given the different tasks Dr Steven was attempting to perform at the same time in her immunisation clinic it was felt that errors were inevitable.

Dr Steven's honesty in describing her error resulted in two tangible benefits. She returned to her own practice determined to make changes in the way her immunisation clinics were organised and serviced by practice staff. Armed with the constructive practical suggestions from her colleagues she was confident that changes could be implemented in her own practice. The discussion group itself also benefited from her initiative. A group that was in danger of disintegrating found new enthusiasm by being able to tackle a sensitive issue in an honest and supportive manner.

Neither the mother nor the baby was upset by the additional injection!

Neither of these two examples concerns life threatening problems. Fortunately such events are rare in general practice. The lessons that can be learnt from the recognition of clinical mistakes, however, do not depend on the seriousness of the clinical consequences. Indeed it may be easier to learn from less serious mistakes because blame and feelings of guilt are less likely to impede analysis of the factors involved than is the case for serious mistakes.

General practice is an operational specialty. Clinical mistakes are likely to involve organisational factors as well as pure clinical medicine. Indeed the identification of administrative errors is an excellent starting point for auditing practice organisation and will be considered further in the chapter on auditing the organisation.

Conclusion

Learning from the audit of clinically significant events is endless. The events that I have considered are just examples from the wide range of clinical material that is available. Further examples are considered in the chapter on auditing the organisation, because the audit of clinical events often reveals organisational as well as medical problems.

In this chapter I have tried to be positive and provocative about medical audit. The future of general practice will be bleak if audit is seen to be a mechanical process of data collection within a system that penalises deviations from the norm. I began the chapter by stating that the audit of clinically significant events raises more questions than answers. Audits should be cyclical activities in which structured inquiry leads to a deeper understanding of the processes of care and to the formulation of better questions and better ways of collecting information. Research and audit are sometimes considered to be separate activities, but good audit projects lead to questions that can be researched and are of general relevance.

1 New Leeuwenhorst Group. *Quality improvement by quality assessment—a first statement.* Amsterdam: Huisarten Instituut Vinje Universiteit Amsterdam, 1986.
2 Pendleton D (ed). *The consultation: an approach to learning and teaching.* Oxford: Oxford University Press, 1984.
3 Byrne P, Long BEL. *Doctors talking to patients.* London: Royal College of General Practitioners, 1976.
4 Stott N, Davis RH. The exceptional potential in each primary care consultant. *J R Coll Gen Pract* 1979;**29**:201–5.

Further reading
Anonymous. Critical questions; critical incidents; critical answers. *Lancet* 1988;**i**:1373–4.
Newble DI. The critical incident technique: a new approach to the assessment of clinical performance. *Medical Education* 1983;**167**:401–30.

7 The audit of prescribing

MARSHALL MARINKER,
JACQUELINE V JOLLEYS

Introduction

The audit of prescribing should not be seen as an end in itself. The appropriateness of the prescription relates to the appopriateness of the diagnosis on which it is based. In general practice many diagnoses cannot be elaborated beyond the level of symptoms. Even when the symptoms and other information lead to a diagnosis, that diagnosis may simply be a reformulation of the symptoms, rather than a statement about antecedent causes. Further, successful diagnosis and treatment demand adequate communication with the patient, because without understanding compliance is unlikely. In short, the audit of prescribing provides us with a window on the audit of the whole clinical process. Consequently a modern general practice might determine the following:

- That drugs are only prescribed in relation to a defensible formulation of the patient's problems
- That the simplest regimen is selected to achieve the optimum result
- That the optimum medication is achieved at minimum cost.

In pursuit of this, the practice would create a system in which:

- Prescribing is routinely monitored in relation to individual patients, individual doctors, and the performance of the practice.

The need to audit prescribing in the NHS has long been recognised. Although, by international comparison, the expenditure

116

on drugs in the NHS is comparatively modest, the cost of prescribing increases year by year, and it represents an increasing proportion of total NHS costs. There is also a range of variation in the prescribing levels of doctors which cannot be explained solely in terms of variations in morbidity between practice populations, but seems to be a reflection of the idiosyncratic choices of individual doctors. The task of relating these individual variations to the quality of care is one of the true goals of medical audit. It is, however, understandable perhaps that it is the increase and variations in cost that concern Government.

For this reason, long before the term "medical audit" became fashionable, and before medical audit became a required activity in modern general practice, *the Prescription Pricing Authority* (PPA) had been auditing general practice prescribing. The aim was clearly cost containment.

At the time of writing, data on prescribing analyses and cost (PACT) provide an increasingly detailed feedback of prescribing levels and costs to the individual doctor, and to the practice. Although the avowed intention is to improve the quality of decision making about prescribing, and not simply to contain cost, PACT data are primarily concerned with quantities, distributions, and price. The description of PACT, and its role in the audit of prescribing, are given in the Appendix to this chapter.

Essentially data of this sort are comparative. This means that the feedback expresses volumes of prescribing, quantities, distributions, and costs in relation to averages—practice averages, locality averages, and national averages. Although statements about quantities, averages, distributions, and comparisons are not in themselves indications of appropriateness or quality, they may be presented as proxies for quality judgments based on the questionable notion that averages represent some sort of professional consensus. In fact averages represent no such consensus, and they do not constitute a desired standard. The successful audit of prescribing, as for all medical audit, should relate not to more or less arbitrary averages of performance, but to the best evidence available about optimum care.

A report of the Health Select Committee[1] in 1994 came to the conclusion that a rationally prescribed drug would have been chosen in relation to:

- Effectiveness
- Safety

- Convenience (relative to other drugs or other forms of treatment)
- Cost (when the previous criteria have been satisfied).

The first of these three desiderata is concerned with notions of quality and relates to best practice, the results of clinical research, health economics, and so on. The fourth relates to the statistical analysis of peer behaviour, to expenditure targets, and to constraints, and in itself gives no direct indication of the achievement of desired standards of care. Today it is widely recognised that the auditing of prescribing is concerned primarily with achieving these desired standards.

A framework for audit

In this chapter a framework for rational audit is suggested under the following eight headings:

- Evidence of underprescribing
- Evidence of overprescribing
- The choice of effective drug
- The choice of effective regimen
- Monitoring for costs
- The relationship between cost and benefit
- Compliance
- Learning from errors.

Evidence of underprescribing

Hitherto underprescribing has received far less attention than overprescribing. By underprescribing is meant an absence or relatively low level of prescribing of a particular drug or class of drugs, in relation to the expected prevalence of certain chronic conditions in the practice population.

A simple example concerns the therapeutic response to children who present with cough. In the past much attention has been given to the appropriateness or inappropriateness of prescribing antibiotics for children with upper respiratory tract infections. This may not, however, be the most relevant prescribing issue here. Doctors in a group practice may be invited to record their prescriptions when responding to children who present with cough, or where cough is one of the major components of the complaint. If the records of such children between the ages of three and 10 years are examined, there may be an interesting variation between partners in the level of prescribing of asthma related drugs. This may indicate that those doctors who prescribe very few or no such drugs in this situation may be ignoring the fact that persistent or recurrent cough in children is one of the common ways in which asthma presents.

It is essential that these data are collected from *consecutive* consultations carried out by each doctor. If the audit takes place at a time of year when upper respiratory tract infections are rife, each doctor may be able to provide evidence from some 10 or 20 patients—enough to give some sense of his or her prescribing habit. Although this audit cannot be regarded as quantitatively adequate, it is in fact a useful qualitative audit, the results of which raise important questions about appropriate diagnosis.

Any prescribing profile in which there is an absence, or very low level, of prescribing in relation to expected morbidities deserves close inspection. Examples would include the absence of: dual or triple therapy for patients with chronic peptic ulcer; angiotensin converting enzyme (ACE) inhibitors for patients with heart failure; antihypertensive or antidepressant treatment; or appropriate therapy in postmyocardial infarction patients.

Evidence of overprescribing

This refers not to errors of regimen (dealt with later), but rather to the tendency to prescribe where it would be more appropriate not to. The starting point may legitimately be comparative data: an examination of outlying high prescribers.[1] Examples would include: high levels of long term prescribing of hypnotics and anxiolytics; the non-intermittent prescribing of non-steroidal anti-inflammatory drugs (NSAIDs); the routine use of high potency steroid dermatological preparations; and the routine use of antibiotics or drugs to control the symptoms of minor upper respiratory tract infections.

The choice of effective drug

For the most part doctors are taught that there are substantial advantages in using older, tested, and tried remedies rather than the latest innovations. From the point of view of safety there is much sense in this, because the use of these older preparations is supported by a great weight of data over very many years. From the point of view of cost, also, this makes sense. Older preparations are no longer protected by patent, and their generic equivalents are often cheaper than the original proprietary brands.

Many innovations, however, do in fact confer substantial benefit. Where this has been established, the use of older preparations must be questioned. Examples could be found in the modern management of heart failure, postmyocardial infarction, migraine, peptic ulcer, and so on, where failure to offer the patient newer and more expensive preparations may actually be negligent. Auditing for effective medication is probably best done by the consecutive review of records of patients who have these and other chronic diseases where therapeutic advances have been particularly important in recent years.

The choice of effective regimen

For most chronic conditions most drugs are best introduced in relatively low doses, and the dose then built up to the optimum for the patient and the disease. An exception is the prescription of some drugs in acute exacerbations of chronic diseases—for example, the introduction of high doses of steroids in status asthmaticus. Much may be learned by an examination of a series of records from patients with, for example, high blood pressure or depression. Where the response to poorly controlled blood pressure and depression is routinely to change the medication every few weeks, rather than to attempt to titrate the dose, it would be helpful to review this prescribing technique.

The duration of medication for many chronic conditions sometimes needs to be lifelong. Medication often needs, however, to be time limited or "pulsed," or limited to the duration of an exacerbation. Examples include the use of NSAIDs in osteoarthritis, H_2-receptor antagonists in a variety of causes of dyspepsia, oral steroids in Crohn's disease, bronchodilators in asthma, and antibiotics in exacerbations of chronic obstructive airway disease.

In relation to each of these and other similar conditions, an audit can reveal whether the prescribing approach is standardised and insensitive to the natural history of the condition and the response of the patient, or constantly monitored so that, although the optimum medication is given, the prescribing is appropriately intermittent or varied.

Monitoring for safety

The decision to prescribe any drug involves a judgment about the balance between the desired benefits and the danger (however

120

small) of damage. The more serious the potential damage, the greater the need for vigilance—even though the incidence of this damage may be expected to be low. Audit should be aimed to reflect the level of such vigilance. Examples include: an annual check of thyroid stimulating hormone in the case of patients receiving thyroxine; the monitoring of serum urea and electrolytes in patients receiving diuretics, whose renal function is already compromised; and appropriate blood testing when the required drug is known to be capable of suppressing bone marrow (for example, mianserin in depressive illness).

The more serious the condition and the greater the likelihood of therapeutic benefit, the more the patient may be willing, and the doctor deem it prudent, to take risks. It is not easy to audit the quality of a doctor's ethical thinking in this regard. If the practice is in the habit of reviewing video taped consultations, however, attention might be paid to the frequency with which the relationship between benefit and risk is discussed with the patient.

Known incompatibilities and contraindications should also be monitored. For example, audit should alert the general practitioner to the prescription of NSAIDs for patients with obstructive airway disease or peptic ulceration. Much may be learned from the analysis of errors (see the discussion of confidential inquiries below). A practice policy of inquiring into all prescribing "accidents" would, in itself, provide an important mechanism for risk avoidance.

The relationship between cost and benefit

Quite apart from pressures from Government sources to contain the cost of prescribing, there is clearly an ethical imperative to contain cost—consonant with achieving optimum effectiveness. The prescriber has a public duty to use NHS resources as efficiently as possible. In most cases the cost of proprietary drugs is greater than that of their generic equivalents, and such differences in bioavailability as may exist are not by and large clinically important. For this reason, a practice policy of generic prescribing, when the choice exists, makes sense. An audit of prescribing will soon pick up deviations from this policy. Such deviations, of course, are not in themselves judgments about the inappropriateness of the prescription. They simply question it. There may be all sorts of reasons concerned with patient preference and compliance, for example, which may justify the continuation of a proprietary medicine, and the decision not to switch to a generic alternative. Audit ensures, however, that the question is asked.

By the same token, because generic pills and capsules may come in a variety of different shapes, sizes, and colours, it may be deemed prudent to prescribe a known proprietary drug for a confused patient, so that the appearance will not vary from one prescription to another. As with all medical audit, deviations from an agreed norm or guideline should, in the first instance, provoke inquiry rather than adverse comment.

There is no gold standard of cost–benefit analysis. The cost of medicines may be judged in relation to the biotechnical outcome, and this in turn may relate to the cost of the patient's incapacity—the financial consequences of withholding the medication or of choosing an alternative. Health economists might include a whole range of potential benefits in relation to the cost of medication: possible savings on hospitalisation and the more expensive treatment modalities that might follow from this; the long term consequences of inadequately controlled symptoms, of unemployment, of informal caring; and much else.

Considerations such as these cannot enter into the equation of the individual doctor's choice about his or her individual patient in any quantifiable way. They may, perhaps they must, however, influence the quality of the doctor's thinking about cost and benefit. In practical terms, for the general practitioner the choice is between generic and proprietary preparations, and between competing proprietary preparations, when the cheapest effective drug is evidently the most defensible first choice.

Compliance

Compliance is an important issue, even if the term "compliance" is an unfortunate one. It carries with it overtones of professional paternalism and of a failure to respect the autonomy of the individual patient. The term "non-compliance" seems to imply a criticism of the patient, as though failure to follow doctor's orders results from moral turpitude, or at best from ignorance and stupidity. In fact compliance depends on a number of quite complex issues:

- A mismatch of health beliefs—the patient's understanding of the doctor's beliefs, and the doctor's of the patient's

- The doctor's skills in communication
- The quality of the doctor/patient relationship.

Failures of compliance may result from the following:

- A confusional state (even mild, and occasionally brought on by the very drugs that the doctor has already prescribed)
- A failure to understand the purposes of the medication and the benefits of adherence to the recommended regimen
- The patient's unwillingness, therefore, to tolerate the unwanted effects of medication
- A conscious decision to reject the doctor's diagnosis and/or not to cooperate with the treatment.

For the most part issues of compliance are raised when repeat prescriptions are audited.[2] Failures to pick up repeat prescriptions, or the request for fresh prescriptions much earlier than expected, should alert the practice to some problems with compliance. Much more frequently problems of compliance may become evident from the audit of the individual case. These require the techniques of confidential inquiry.

Learning from errors

In chapter 1 of this book the importance of auditing individual cases is argued, and in chapter 2 a framework for confidential inquiries (REPOSE) is described. Errors arising from prescribing provide a very important opportunity in general practice. They are more reliably identified when they are actively sought. Further, if they are actively sought they are likely to be caught at an earlier stage in the problem. Very old people, and patients with confusional states, are particularly vulnerable. The following is an incomplete list of opportunities to search for errors and to institute such inquiries:

- Any failures in the repeat prescription system
- Any examples of morbidity resulting from non-compliance
- Random audit of patients who may be confused because of age, disease, social isolation, or multiple medication
- A review of medication (not only what is prescribed but what remains in bathroom cabinets) when an elderly patient becomes ill, requests a home visit, or is admitted as an emergency to hospital.

Conclusion

Franz Kafka wrote "To write prescriptions is easy, but to come to an understanding with people is hard." To write rational prescriptions is not always easy, and in general practice it would be true to say that it is impossible to prescribe rationally without coming to an understanding with the patient. As this chapter has sought to suggest, a vigorous approach to the audit of prescribing can illuminate the quality of individual clinical problem solving, the quality of the relationship between doctor and patient, and the efficiency of the practice organisation in serving these ends.[3]

Appendix

Prescribing analysis and costs (PACT)

Prescribing analysis and costs or PACT consists of a set of reports. These inform general practitioners (GPs) about their prescribing in terms of cost over the preceding three month period. The data in the reports—generated by the Prescription Pricing Authority (PPA)—give information about drugs and appliances that have been prescribed by the individual doctor and by his or her practice as a whole; these prescribing costs are then compared with those of other GPs in the same Family Health Services Authority (FHSA) and with the level of costs nationally. The reports are presented as a series of tables, histograms, and graphs. These enable practitioners to see whether the costs attributable to their practice are high, average, or low.

PACT is available at two levels:

1 The PACT Standard Report which is sent to all GPs and practices automatically
2 A more detailed PACT Prescribing Catalogue available on request.

PACT Standard Report

This report describes the practice's prescribing practices, comparing them with those of other GPs in the same FHSA. It points out those therapeutic areas that have relatively high costs for the practice and also indicates the contributions of the individual GPs to that cost. Costs are broken down into six major therapeutic groups of costs; in addition the report lists the 20 most expensive drugs used by the practice, highlighting new drugs and those available as generic formulations.

One criticism of PACT's Standard Report is that it does not take into account any demographic variables. In fact it uses only prescribing units in adjusting the information to the number of elderly patients in the practice.

PACT Prescribing Catalogue

If the practice wish to look at their prescribing patterns in more detail—and this is necessary for conducting a full audit—then they need to request a PACT Prescribing Catalogue. This report gives a detailed summary of general practitioners' prescribing within the given time period. The information is broken down into the subheadings of the *British National Formulary*. This information is again compared with the average prescribing within the practice's FHSA.

PACT Indicative Prescribing Scheme Catalogue

There is a third report available; this comprises a cumulative catalogue that is useful for monitoring the use that the practice makes of its formulary. It also looks at the trends that occur in prescribing.

1 Audit Commission. *A prescription for improvement. Towards more rational prescribing in General Practice.* London: HMSO, 1994.
2 Department of Health. *National Audit Office: Repeat prescribing by general medical practitioners in England.* Executive letter EL(93)73, 1993.
3 Pringle M, Bradley C, *et al. Significant event auditing.* Occasional Paper 70. London: Royal College of General Practitioners, 1995.

8 Managing the practice for quality

BRENDA SAWYER, ROSEY FOSTER,
SANDRA GOWER

The 1990s have heralded the age of the Charter—the Citizen's Charter, the Patient's Charter, the Parents' Charter—and practices are now being encouraged to compile a personalised version. Patients have been made more aware of their rights and doctors their responsibilities; there must also be greater accountability in general medical practice. In the 1980s the move towards total quality management started; in the current decade we are seeing the benefits and necessity of implementing audit.

What has this meant for the organisation and management of practice? How do we audit the management of the practice? In fact, no audit of the individual or the organisation should be done in isolation, but should rather involve the whole practice team.

In this chapter we explore different methods of evaluating the management and the organisation of the practice, share some of the experiences of those who are taking part, and look at other bodies that influence practices to undertake quality audit.

Total quality management

The concept of total quality management became increasingly important during the 1980s. Ron Collard in his book *Total quality: success through people*[1] describes the challenge that this concept presents to management: he stresses the importance of people, the need for involvement of all concerned, and for training. In his book six fundamental requirements are listed:

- Commitment from top management
- Change of attitude
- Continuous improvement
- Strengthened supervision
- Extensive training
- Recognition of improvement.

To meet these requirements it is obvious that there is a need for audit, but not just of the individual. In his book *Managing for quality in general practice*,[2] Donald Irvine recognises that doctors have been wary of broadening the audit of quality from auditing the performance of individuals, that is, clinical audit, to a wider context of consideration—for example, patient satisfaction. Should change be the result of the audit of clinical performance as perceived by doctors, or should it be the result of performance of the practice as seen by the Family Health Services Authority (FHSA)? Irvine explores the need for accountability and the concepts of quality: "Quality is about working together." It is vital to foster relationships when dealing with quality—quality is a collective mindset which is attained through people's links with each other. In the commercial world, we speak of the chain of suppliers and customers: everyone, including every team, is a supplier to someone and a customer of someone else. This is the key to quality.[3] The concept of the customer, whether external or internal, is integral to a total quality approach. External customers are all those who are not employed by the practice, that is, patients, hospitals, FHSAs, etc; internal customers would include staff, most of whom, in their turn, would be relying on other staff to help in the fulfilment of the service to the external customer. For example, a receptionist may require the general practitioner to sign prescriptions rapidly so that patients' scripts are ready for collection when they arrive—the receptionist is the internal customer of the general practitioner. Likewise, partners in a practice will require their appointment system to work effectively, by having the notes readily available for the correct patient—the partners are the internal customers of the receptionist who has the role of preparing the surgeries.

Everyone in the practice is working ultimately to fulfil the needs of the end customer, the patient. Satisfying the needs of the internal customer is a vital interim step. Individuals need to help each other to perform their role well to the overall benefit of the practice.[4]

The need for involvement of the whole team has started to be accepted, as can be seen from recently published documents. The

127

NHS Management Executive's Collation of Evaluative Projects 1991–3[5] explores the impact of audit on patient care, stating that "the range of practice team members involved in audit is getting wider, topics audited are becoming more appropriate, audit skills are improving and interest in audit has increased." It suggests that large, well organised practices are more likely to be carrying out audit because resources are scarcer for smaller practices. It also identifies practices with computerisation and a practice manager as being more likely to be involved, so these are some of the influential factors in the decision to undertake audit.

The *A–Z of quality* published by the NHS Executive[6] describes two projects concerned with implementing total quality management in primary care.

The first involved four general practices in Dorset and Wiltshire, which defined total quality management as involving:

- management leadership
- organisation wide implementation
- everyone being responsible for quality
- continuous improvement
- a clear purpose
- shared values, with a patient centred approach.

It is interesting that great emphasis was placed on the concept of "understanding what team working means" and how this could benefit the delivery of primary care involving the practice. A structured approach was adopted with the model of action centred learning. The project was carefully monitored and key issues were agreed for improvements to quality. Each practice produced a report detailing the steps that needed to be taken for the implementation of changes.

The second project, also using the model of total quality management, concentrated on the relationship between the practice and its patients. By using patient feedback on services, necessary improvements could be identified, whether within the practice, at the interface of practice and patient, or at the interface of primary and secondary care.

Vocational training scheme for general practitioners

The vocational training regulations laid down in 1979 established that no new entrant to general practice could become a principal without undergoing a three year training programme; of this one year was spent in an approved training practice. To become an approved training practice, a considerable amount of audit needs to be carried out for assessing where the practice meets the regional criteria and where improvement is needed. Not only is the general practitioner trainer assessed, but also the standard of the practice, which effectively means that the total quality of the practice is examined.

Three important areas in the organisation of the practice are closely examined and assessed: the state of medical records, medical equipment, and the practice library. The records must be legible, tidy, in order, with a summary insert. There should also be a disease and age–sex register. The library must contain relevant, easily accessible books available for the trainee and partners. It would be usual for a training practice to have an ECG machine and other medical equipment. It is probable that the trainee will have had the opportunity of using such equipment in the hospital environment. Most training practices will, however, now be computerised so it may be necessary to assess the current skills, if any, of the trainee to identify appropriate training needs for effective use of computers.

The National Joint Committee for Post-Graduate Training For General Practice devolves the responsibility for assessment to the regions; in each region there is a Regional GP Education Committee, and the regional adviser, who is the executive officer of that Committee, is responsible for all general practitioner training in that region. It is the regional adviser, or representative, who leads the formal visit to assess the suitability of a practice as a training practice.

It is usually the manager in practice who does much of the work in coordinating the audit of the organisation, helping to identify improvements needed, and implementing any changes. The manager often liaises about the necessary arrangements for the assessment visit, so there must be a high standard of management skills in the practice.

Individual audit of management skills

National Vocational Qualifications

Marshall Marinker refers to clinical standards in chapter 2, and this is an appropriate starting point to explore the possibilities of

129

measuring quality in the non-clinical areas. A pivotal person in the organisation is usually the manager(s). In the growing practice team there may be more than one person undertaking managerial responsibilities, for example, a practice nurse manager, a fund manager, a business manager, a finance manager, and the general practitioners. It is now possible to measure competence against a nationally agreed and recognised set of management standards. In the past we have relied heavily on academic qualifications, on the acquisition of knowledge, rather than assessing whether a person is able to perform effectively in the real world.

In 1985 a review body was set up by the Government to review the acceptability of vocational qualifications in England and Wales. The committee reported back in 1986 recommending that a new organisation be set up to implement its findings. This became the National Council for Vocational Qualifications (NCVQ). Their main aim was to devise qualifications relevant to the world of work, enabling progression through to managerial and professional levels. Standards were to be developed for all occupations and were to apply across all occupational sectors. These qualifications are called National Vocational Qualifications (NVQs). The key criterion for an NVQ is that it must be based on standards required for the workplace. These standards are devised by Lead Bodies which are made up of employers who are recognised as representing the needs and views of its Sector members.

The Management Charter Initiative

In 1988 the Management Charter Initiative (MCI) was formed with its aim to improve the performance of organisations in the United Kingdom through improvement in the quality of managers. The three foundation partners were the CBI (Confederation of British Industry), the BIM (British Institute of Management), and the Foundation for Management Education, under the chairmanship of Sir Bob Reid, with backing from organisations, including Shell, IBM, BP, and the Government. In 1990 the MCI was nominated by the Government as the lead body responsible for developing management standards. During the period between 1989 and 1992, this forum conducted nationwide research to develop the management standards. Over 4000 managers were questioned to identify the key roles and levels of management performance required by managers. Those questioned came from the private, public, and voluntary sectors of small, medium, and large organisations. From this research it was possible to identify the various levels of managers at different stages in their careers—the performance criteria, the underpinning knowledge, understanding, and the personal effectiveness needed for a manager to be competent. Four distinctive levels were identified for managers at different stages: supervisory managers, first line managers, middle managers, and senior managers.

Supervisory managers—They do not take full control or responsibility for activities, but they do contribute to management activities, although the first line manager has the full responsibility for these.

First line managers—They have a limited span of control but are responsible for certain defined areas of activity and of using resources effectively and efficiently. This includes managing people and monitoring progress of the practice against set objectives.

Middle managers—Although these managers do not have responsibility for strategic management of the practice, they do have a greater span of control and responsibility than first line managers, and this brings with it a high degree of accountability. They play a significant part in the management of change and development of the organisation.

Senior managers—These provide leadership for their organisation, and are responsible for strategic development and implementation.

In general practice these four levels become the following:

1 *Supervisory manager*—a senior receptionist who contributes to some management activities and reports to a manager.
2 *First line manager*—a manager who implements practice policy set by the partners and has responsibility for certain areas of the practice, but reports to the partnership.
3 *Middle manager*—a manager who is an equal with the partners, albeit not necessarily a legal partner, but with an equal vote and voice, contributing to the policy and decision making of the partnership.
4 *Senior manager*—a manager of a consortium or a primary health care team.

131

There are three sets of standards that have been published for middle managers (M2), first line managers (M1), and supervisory managers (MIS), and the draft standards for senior managers (M3) are at the trial stage. In addition, a model on personal competence, or effectiveness, has also been produced. This recognises the role that personal behaviour plays in effective management performance.

The Association of Managers in General Practice (AMGP) initiated a project gathering examples of evidence from general medical practice; this project was to provide proof of competence against the performance criteria set for the Management Level I Standards for the first line manager. These have been published jointly by the Association, the National Health Service Training Division of the National Health Service Executive, and CIBA Pharmaceuticals. A research project is under way which is examining whether or not the implementation of management standards in general practice makes any difference to the quality of patient care.

The standards

The MCI describes the concept of competence as "the ability of a manager to perform to the standards required in employment."[6] The standards describe what managers need to do if they are doing their jobs competently, and are divided into four bands called key roles: (1) manage operations; (2) manage finance; (3) manage people; and (4) manage information.

The individual skills of personal competence are a necessary part of achieving effective competence in carrying out a job, and these skills include the ability to plan, to manage others, to manage yourself, and to use your intellect, that is, a personal competence model can describe the personal behaviour needed to perform effectively. In addition managers need to have an underlying knowledge and understanding of the practice as a whole to perform competently.

Structure of the management standards (fig 8.1)

The four key roles can be broken down into *units* of competence; these explain what is expected of competent managers in particular areas of their job. The units are divided into *elements* which reflect in greater detail the necessary skills, knowledge, and understanding. Elements, in turn, contain a number of *performance criteria* which

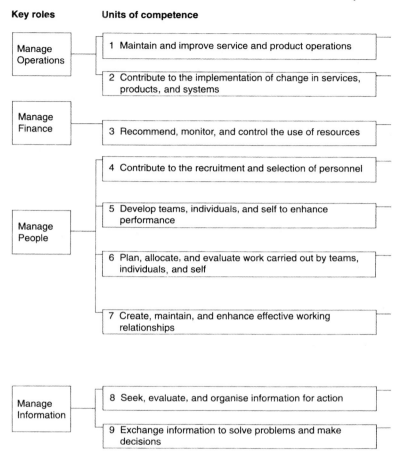

Key roles

Units of competence

Manage Operations

1 Maintain and improve service and product operations

2 Contribute to the implementation of change in services, products, and systems

Manage Finance

3 Recommend, monitor, and control the use of resources

4 Contribute to the recruitment and selection of personnel

5 Develop teams, individuals, and self to enhance performance

Manage People

6 Plan, allocate, and evaluate work carried out by teams, individuals, and self

7 Create, maintain, and enhance effective working relationships

Manage Information

8 Seek, evaluate, and organise information for action

9 Exchange information to solve problems and make decisions

Fig 8.1—Overview of the first line management standards. (Reproduced from First Line Management Standards—Level I, the Management Charter Initiative)

can be used as the basis for collecting the necessary evidence for assessment of a manager's competence. *Range indicators* describe the situations in which personal competence is needed. Description of sources and types of *evidence* provides some examples that can be used in the process of assessing competence.

Use of management standards in general practice

Three broad areas describe the main benefits of using management standards.

133

Elements of competence

1.1 Maintain operations to meet quality of standards
1.2 Create and maintain the necessary conditions for productive work

2.1 Contribute to the evaluation of proposed changes to services, products, and systems
2.2 Implement and evaluate changes to services, products, and systems

3.1 Make recommendations for expenditure
3.2 Monitor and control the use of resources

4.1 Define future personnel requirements
4.2 Contribute to the assessment and selection of candidates against team and organisational requirements

5.1 Develop and improve teams through planning and activities
5.2 Identify, review, and improve development activities for individuals
5.3 Develop oneself with the job role

6.1 Set and update work objectives for teams and individuals
6.2 Plan activities and determine work methods to achieve objectives
6.3 Allocate work and evaluate teams, individuals, and self against objectives
6.4 Provide feedback to teams and individuals on their performance

7.1 Establish and maintain the trust and support of one's subordinates
7.2 Establish and maintain the trust and support of one's immediate manager
7.3 Establish and maintain relationships with colleagues
7.4 Identify and minimise interpersonal conflict
7.5 Implement disciplinary and grievance procedures
7.6 Counsel staff

8.1 Obtain and evaluate information to aid decision making
8.2 Record and store information

9.1 Lead meetings and group discussions to solve problems and make decisions
9.2 Contribute to discussions to solve problems and make decisions
9.3 Advise and inform others

Fig 8.1—*contd.*

Development—A plan of development needs can be compiled by comparing existing competence with management standards. This will identify the areas in which development needs to be implemented.

Design—In identifying the developmental needs, it will become evident where there is a need for training, and a training programme can be designed.

Assessment—In carrying out the above, the standards are providing the means of assessment.

More specifically, the management standards are the basis of National Vocational Qualifications and Scottish Vocational Qualifications for management and supervision. They provide the means of compiling a job description—not only for a practice manager, but also for a manager carrying out specific functions in the practice, such as a finance manager or business development manager, or perhaps for someone who is concerned mainly with managing the staff team.

During the recruitment and selection process the standards can be used as an assessment tool in the comparison of the competence of the applicants, and also in the determination of promotion within a team.

One of the most important functions of effectively managing people is that of appraisal—auditing performance. It is essential that all members of the team have the opportunity for effective and positive appraisal of their performance. The management standards are an objective resource tool which can be used as the basis for this process. Objective measurement is necessary if performance review is to be related to pay. Assessment of levels of competence against the performance criteria provides the opportunity for discussion; and through the personal competence model behaviour and attitude can be explored. This can be used to set targets for future development and planning of the form this development could take. The changes occurring in the NHS demand the use of different skills in the management of general practice, and these skills can be identified from the standards. In some cases existing managers may have the necessary skills for this development although in others it may be necessary to bring in someone else. The standards should therefore be used to construct a new organisational structure.

Fellowship by assessment

In 1990 fellowship by assessment was introduced by the Royal College of General Practitioners; this has been termed the "ultimate audit." In the preface of Occasional Paper 50,[8] Professor Denis Pereira Gray wrote:

Fellowship provides a nationally agreed, uniform set of standards backed up by research evidence and has focused the College's central concern for patients within an organisation framework . . .

Fellowship is open to every member of the college who has been in active practice for five years and who can provide formal written evidence that they have achieved the standard of patient care as delivered and published by the college. Age is not a criterion and fellowship can be achieved by 33 years of age.

There are 16 specific areas and a total of 67 essential criteria to prepare and achieve before the applicant receives an assessment visit by three external assessors, all appointed by the college. One of these assessors is normally from the local faculty to ensure an understanding of the practice's local circumstances.

The areas of care specified by the criteria are those in the box.

The doctor

Entry requirements, accessibility, clinical services, the consultation, other communication skills, performance review, personal qualities, and postgraduate education

The partnership

The practice, staff, library, and practice information

The profession

Medical activities, writing, services to society, and services to the College

---

Preparation for assessment cannot be achieved in isolation and teamwork is central to achieving success. Although this "ultimate audit" may seem to be unachievable to many general practitioners compulsory reaccreditation is becoming a reality for the profession, an issue that can no longer be avoided and one that, in the future, will affect every member of the primary health care team.

We started with an examination of the means of ensuring that the practice is effectively managed—a way that enables the management of the organisation to be audited through a powerful resource tool and to develop the skills of management within practice. Fellowship by assessment, although containing a large element of individual audit, extends to include the whole practice and so leads us to explore more specific ways of auditing the whole team.

Audit of the team

Investors in People UK

The National Training Task Force (NTTF) was set up by the "Employment for the 1990s" white paper which was given two tasks:

1 To set up a network of Training and Enterprise Councils (TECs)
2 To develop a strategy to encourage employers to increase their commitment to train and develop their workforce.

Over a period of 6–9 months working groups developed the strategy which was used to set the standard. A number of "good" employers were used taken from a variety of successful organisations from all sectors. Work done by the Department of Employment's initiative with employers, such as National Training Awards and Business Growth Training, was also used.

During this period the CBI had formed a task force, led by Sir Bryan Nicholson, and they were looking at similar issues. As their report, "Towards a Skills Revolution," reached similar conclusions it was decided that the two should be combined. Thus the national standard was launched in November 1990 by Michael Howard, Secretary of State for Employment.

The national "Standard for Effective Investment in People"[9] contains four principles: commitment, review, action, and evaluation. The aim is to encourage and recognise effective training and development, where effective training is training that is strategically planned and linked to business objectives, and will improve business performance. A more detailed description is given below.

The national standard of an "Investor in People" is that they "make a public commitment from the top to develop all employees to achieve its business objectives." In other words, general practitioners and their managers who have set aims and objectives for their practices ensure that all members of their team know what is expected of them in contributing to the provision of patient care. How can this be implemented and assessed? The set of standards—assessment indicators—can be used by TECs (Local

Enterprise Companies (LECs) in Scotland) to ascertain whether the practice can be recognised as an Investor in People. These standards apply to small and large, public and private organisations. Although it is possible to gain an award for the practice—an event that can motivate the whole team—it is also possible to use the standards simply to assess and develop individuals.

Principal standards—There are four principal standards for an Investor in People. The first is a public commitment from the top to develop the ability of all employees to achieve its business objectives:

- Every employer should have a written, although flexible, plan which sets out business goals and targets, considers how employees will contribute to achieving the plan, and specifies how development needs in particular will be assessed and met
- Management should develop and communicate to all employees a vision of where the organisation is going and the contribution employees will make to its success, involving employee representatives as appropriate.

The second standard is the regular review of the training and development needs of all employees:

- The resources for training and developing employees should be clearly identified in the business plan
- Managers should be responsible for agreeing training and development needs with each employee on a regular basis, in the contexts of business objectives, setting targets, and linking standards, where appropriate, to the achievement of National Vocational Qualifications (or relevant units)—in Scotland, Scottish Vocational Qualifications.

The third standard is to take action in the training and development of individuals when they are recruited and throughout their employment:

- Action should focus on the training needs of all new recruits and the continual development and improvement of the skills of existing employees
- All employees should be encouraged to contribute to identifying and meeting their own job related development needs.

The fourth standard is the evaluation of the investment in training and development to assess achievement and improve future effectiveness:

- The investment, the competence, and commitment of employees, and the use made of skills learnt, should be reviewed at all levels against business goals and targets
- The effectiveness of training and development should be reviewed at the top level and lead to renewed commitment and target setting.

These four broad areas can be further broken down into *assessment indicators* which describe more specifically what is expected.

The partnership must be fully, and openly, committed to developing the potential of everyone in their team. To meet these standards successfully, it is necessary to have a very detailed and clear business plan stating the aims and objectives of the practice so that achievement can be assessed easily. Specific practice goals and targets must be indicated, together with the methods used for assessing whether these goals have been met. Communication with all members of the team must be effective, with a clear indication of those involved in meeting the specific targets; it should be borne in mind that it is important for representative members of the teams, such as the nursing team and the reception team, to be involved in this process.

The business plan has to identify the resources necessary to meet the training and development needs of the team, and these needs must be reviewed regularly against practice objectives and individual employee's needs. Managers have to have the skills suitable for carrying out these assessments and for the fulfilment of the development needs of the organisation as a whole. At every level the individuals responsible must be clearly identified in the business plan, and each individual must be aware of his or her own specific targets and those of the wider team.

Great importance is attached to the induction period for new staff. Implementing assessment of competence and knowledge at the recruitment stage means that the process of development starts at induction. An example is when a new medical secretary has been identified at interview as being competent in word processing but has not used the particular software package used by the

139

practice. It is necessary to plan a suitable method of acquiring knowledge and skills in using the software and this will probably start during the induction period—whether in house by an existing secretary, through reading the manual, practising on the word processor, attending an external training course, watching a training video, or by a combination of some, or all, of these activities. The method and timing of regular review of the competence of new employees need to be discussed and recorded.

General practices are in a state of constant change. In particular, the change of emphasis in the delivery of patient care is having a dramatic effect on the provision of services. The swing from provision in the secondary sector to delivery of more services in primary care has resulted in the need to update the skills of the whole practice team. Business objectives are altering and there is a need to keep all the team informed, and involved, from the earliest stages in the process of change. Change can lead to explosive conflict in a team, and managers will need the competence to deal with the such conflict, and to support team members through crises.

Some changes have led to new opportunities for career progression and it is important that members of staff are aware of these opportunities. It is necessary to provide a framework for continuing review of skills for the identification of developmental needs and to take appropriate actions to meet these needs.

"Investors in People" ensures that evaluation of these development actions has actually achieved the practice objectives.

Organisational audit

The King's Fund Organisational Audit Programme[10]

In 1897 the King Edward's Hospital Fund was founded as the result of an appeal asking the people of London to contribute to a permanent fund. The capital, and the interest that built up following this appeal, was first used to make grants to hospitals. It has, over the years, widened this brief and now seeks to encourage and support the development of services in all areas of health care.

The King's Fund defines organisational audit as:

> . . . a national approach to setting and monitoring standards for the organisation of health care services. The standards are concerned with the systems and structures which must be in place in order to support

high quality patient/client care. However, standards serve little purpose if there is no objective means of assessing or measuring whether compliance with these is achieved.

The last sentence can be applied to all standards, whether clinical, management, or organisational.

The quality of patient care depends on good clinical practice and on good management, organisation, and delivery of patient services. The Organisational Audit Programme started its activities in the acute sector and the King's Fund report that about one quarter of all acute hospitals in the United Kingdom carry out systematic reviews of the management of their organisations. They extended the Programme to include primary care in January 1994. Further extension into the process for community hospitals is currently under way. The Primary Health Care Programme enables primary health care teams to assess and develop their services.

The process of implementing the King's Fund Organisational Audit Programme starts with its launch to the whole primary health care team, and should include managers from the FHSAs and Community NHS Trusts. This is carried out by a survey manager appointed by the King's Fund. A coordinator is appointed from within the practice and a local steering group is formed.

An initial baseline audit establishes where the standards are met and identifies those areas that need developing. This assessment takes about 4–6 weeks to complete. An action plan and a survey date will then be agreed with the survey manager.

Implementation of the organisational standards usually takes about nine months. The team follow the agreed action plan and six weeks before the survey a self assessment of their compliance with the standards is returned to the survey manager, together with a practice profile. This enables the survey team to have a yardstick against which to measure the primary health care team.

The membership of the survey team is agreed with the primary health care team. Its members will be independent specialists in primary health care, who all undergo specific training for the role of surveyor. The survey usually takes one and a half days. Staff, patients, and users of services are interviewed and the external channels of communication are tested by interviews with FHSA, hospital, and community NHS Trust representatives. Account is taken of the environment, with a review of documentation which provides evidence that policies, procedures, and protocols were followed in practice. Immediate oral feedback of their findings is given by the surveyors.

Six weeks after the survey a confidential, written report is provided by the survey manager incorporating the observations of the surveyors. It presents the positive findings, giving specific commendations for good practice and indicating those areas in which further action is recommended for improvement and change. This enables the primary health care team to formulate an action plan for the continuation of the organisational audit standards for primary health care. Further reviews by the appointed surveyors are carried out at two yearly intervals if the practice continues to subscribe to the programme.

The standards were developed by a central working party, which included people from consumer groups involved in primary care and from professional bodies. Those members of the teams at pilot sites, who were testing the feasibility of the standards, were also involved in their development. There was continual amendment and review by the pilot sites' steering groups and the findings were shared and discussed with the central working group and by consumers. The final manual was published in January 1994. The King's Fund Organisational Audit is now being rolled out to over 50 practices within the United Kingdom.

The standards are divided into four main areas:

1 Core organisational standards and criteria—those that relate to all professionals involved in primary care
2 Professional standards—relating to individual professionals involved in primary care
3 Health records
4 Minor surgery.

The standards have been individually weighted in priority as follows.

Essential practice—If these criteria are not in place, there may be a breach of health and safety or legal regulation, or a compromise of patients' rights.

Good practice—These cover the expected good practice from any primary health care team.

Desirable practice—These cover the criteria that are a means to advancing or improving practice.

Thus the primary health care team is able to establish priorities in meeting the standards and criteria. The King's Fund intends to continue the development of the standards so that, with continual review and update, they comply with current needs.

Two managers from the nine pilot sites identified the main benefits of taking part in this programme as being:

> . . . it provides the framework for a continuous quality improvement programme in practice, thus enabling the Primary Health Care Team to be prepared to meet the challenges of the future.

> . . . it encourages and motivates all members of the Primary Health Care Team to work together effectively as a team, safe in the knowledge that the systems and processes are in place to audit and improve the quality of patient care.

BS 5750

The British standard BS 5750 is a set of national generic standards applicable to quality systems within an organisation. BS 5750 is not a product specification standard, but a management standard system, relating to how quality is provided. It provides a framework of procedures for achieving quality, but it is a means to an end and should not be seen as anything more. It is geared to the achievement of quality of production, not the production of quality.[11]

The standards were initially published in 1979 as the quality assurance standard for manufacturing industries, especially engineering. They were revised in 1987 and harmonised with the International Standard Organisation's ISO 9000 and the European EN 29000 series standards; later they were introduced into the health service and more recently into general practice.

The guiding principle of the standard is the same as that of total quality in general—goods and services are produced right first time.

The emphasis of BS 5750 is on establishing and maintaining an effective quality system, that is, the product or service is designed and delivered in a way that satisfies customer needs. BS 5750 is therefore about systems, when first implementing information technology practices have to:

- Say what they do
- Say why they do it
- Do what they say they will do
- Record what they actually do.[10]

BS 5750 offers processes and is structured in three parts.

Part 1—Standards are related to customer needs and cover such areas as managerial responsibility, the quality system, contract review, design control, document control, purchasing, process control, inspection, testing, measuring and related equipment control of non-conforming products and services, corrective action, handling, storage, packaging and delivering, quality records, training, servicing, and statistical techniques.

Part 2—This is concerned with quality assurance.

Part 3—This is concerned with the final assurance and test stage.

The standard calls for all systems to be documented in considerable detail. Clear, concise, and relevant documentation can be used as a reference to ensure that staff are carrying procedures out correctly. BS 5750 can be used to complement the Investors in People programme.

The benefits of implementing BS 5750 are stated as improving the effectiveness of the organisation. Improved efficiency, time management, and reduction in mistakes should have positive financial implications and lead to improved staff morale and, thus, to a better standard of services and patient care. It is envisaged that a minimum of nine months is needed to implement this quality assurance team.

The standards do not cover continuous development, except by implication, and it requires no specific commitments to employee involvement. The goal of BS 5750 is to pass the test and gain accreditation, whereas other total quality routes search to do things better and improve for continual improvement. Nevertheless the systematic approach can be a good starting point for organisations wishing to start the process of total quality and several general practices have gained the "kite mark."

The Medical Protection Society (MPS) has developed a set of quality assessment guidelines for general practices (GPQA) to

144

assist them in interpreting the requirements of BS 5770 Part 2. Developed and tested within general practice, the manufacturing jargon of BS 5750 has been removed. Each participating practice joins a "GP quality club" and given specialist advice about achieving the quality mark with subsequent monitoring visits. The programme is intended to encourage and foster a "quality" approach to service management in general practice. It does not seek to judge the value of the clinical service provided by the general practitioner but focuses on the organisation and management of the practice and recognises that "the quality of overall health care depends on many factors, not least the efficiency of practice management and the motivation and skill of non-clinical staff." The MPS recognises that when a practice is committed to quality management and continual quality improvement the risks of error, complaints, and mishaps are greatly reduced.

External auditors

Those practices that are fundholding will have been, or will be, depending on when they started, subjected to external audit. This might be by district auditors who examine to check that the systems in place are correct and working effectively, or by representatives from the Audit Commission who have the authority to examine all aspects of the fundholding process including financial records.

Who can help?

Medical Audit Advisory Groups

From April 1991 medical audit became a requirement for practices and Medical Audit Advisory Groups (MAAGs) were set up by FHSAs. Although this is termed "medical audit," it can also include the performance of the practice as a whole, particularly appraisal. Carrying out any audit often involves the managerial, administrative, and clerical members of the team. The MAAGs sometimes provide funding to help with approved audit projects and were set up to stimulate, encourage, and motivate practices to self and peer audit.

Practice Consultancy Programme

None of the routes described is a "quick fix." It requires major cultural change, not inconsiderable financial resources, and

145

commitment over a period of time to generate the energy and enthusiasm needed for the whole team to focus on the route chosen to achieve quality and audit within the practice; even then the process does not stop. As has already been stated, audit is a continuous cycle of improvement and development. But how to start? This can be done by identifying the barriers that prevent effective teamwork and organisation development.

The role of the good consultant adviser, or even of the author of a book on management, is not to say what a practice's goals should be—that is a matter for the health professionals; it is only to help identify and articulate the problems.[11] A joint initiative "Practice Consultancy Programme" of the Royal College of General Practitioners and the Association of Managers in General Practice in 1994, funded by the Department of Health, aims to assist practices in this way. Specially trained primary care professionals will be available for practices to invite to diagnose the blocks and offer possible solutions to effect change.[12]

AMGP "performance review" Diploma module

The Association, as part of its Diploma in Practice Management programme,[14] provides a training module specifically covering performance review. This module can be taken as part of the programme or as a stand alone course. The syllabus includes the principal methods of audit, analysis of information, standard setting, appraisals, and audit of management. The course book is *Managing for quality in general practice* by Donald Irvine.[2]

Although the process of audit may make many demands on resources, both human and financial, the rewards can be motivating. Accreditation by the King's Fund, the award of the "kite mark" for BS 5750, and qualifying for management competence via the NVQ route can all be public demonstrations of achievement, which can be shared with the whole practice team and with patients. The Association of Managers in Practice, with other sponsors, makes an award to the Practice Manager of the Year which gives individual recognition for special achievements.

The future of general practice is changing and challenging. The practice needs to ensure that in the process of change, the quality of services is not compromised. The audit process should be an integral, and continuing, part of every practice's commitment to

146

patient care. "Audit begins by measuring care but its ultimate aim is to improve it."[15]

1 Collard R. *Total quality: success through people.* Institute of Personnel and Development, 1989.
2 Irvine D. *Managing for quality in general practice.* London: The King's Fund Centre, 1990.
3 Wille E. *Quality: achieving excellence.* London: The Sunday Times—Business Skills, 1992.
4 Brooks J, Borgardts I. *Total quality in general practice.* Oxford: Radcliffe Medical Press, 1994.
5 NHS Management Executive. *Medical audit in primary care: a collation of evaluation projects 1991–1993.* London, 1994.
6 *The A–Z of quality: a guide to quality initiatives in the NHS.* London: NHS Management Executive, 1993.
7 Management Charter Initiative. *First line management standards.* London: MCI, 1989.
8 Royal College of General Practitioners. *Occasional paper 50: Fellowship by assessment.* London: RCGP, 1990.
9 Investors in People. *The national standards.* Sheffield: Employment Department, 1991.
10 The King's Fund. *Primary health care organisational standards and criteria manual.* London: The King's Fund, 1994.
11 Irvine S. *Balancing dreams and discipline.* London: RCGP, 1992.
12 BS 5750. *Guidance notes for the application of ISO 9002/EN 29002/BS 5750 Part 2 to general practice.* London: BSI Publications, 1994.
13 *Practice consultancy programme.* RCGP and AMGP, 15 Princes Gate, London SW7 1PU.
14 *AMGP diploma in practice management syllabus.* AMGP, 15 Princes Gate, London SW7 1PU.
15 Crombie IK, Davies HTO, Abraham SCS, Florey du V. *The audit handbook: improving health care through audit.* Chichester: John Wiley & Sons, 1993.

9 The role of the FHSA in medical audit

JONATHAN SHAPIRO

Introduction

It is a truism that many textbooks are out of date by the time they reach the book shops. Even so, there cannot be many chapters in many books that are actually being superseded as they are being written! Yet in spite of the title of this chapter, it is impossible to ignore the fact that Family Health Services Authorities (FHSAs) will disappear by 1996, because legislation combines them with District Health Authorities (DHAs) to form the new Health Authorities.

The name of the organisation is, however, less important than its functions, and in this chapter I hope to discuss the connection between medical audit in primary care and the organisational aspects of the National Health Service in general. I shall describe the evolving nature of medical audit in general practice, its management by FHSAs, and possible future scenarios for managed medical audit. For this, a little background is required concerning the management of general practice over recent years.

Recent history of the management of general practice

FHSAs came into existence in 1990. General practice had until then been under the aegis of the Family Practitioner Committees (FPCs), whose functions were largely clerical. Headed by an administrator, FPCs consisted of a committee of 30 members, about half of whom came from a health professional background. The officers were relatively junior, and their role was to administer general practitioners' nationally negotiated Terms of Service and the fees and allowances.

Thus, the number of general practitioners was set by a national blueprint, item of service payments were monitored by rare and random checks on patients, practice staff reimbursement was allowed up to a maximum of two whole time equivalents per general practitioner, and cost rent schemes were allocated according to nationally determined formulae. The funding required for prescribing was unregulated, and for many years rose in a predictable way which was acceptable to the Treasury of the Government of the moment. Demands were so predictable that funding was not cash limited and, without financial constraints, management was not required.

General practitioners had a contract with FPCs which determined their availability, and a requirement that they would carry out work that was in line with the Terms of Service.

Only a minority of practices, however, monitored consultation rates, prescribing rates, referral rates, immunisation rates, or patient satisfaction.

Part of the reason for this was the real difficulty in actually determining markers of good general practice, a problem that continues to this day. It was, however, mainly to do with the ethos of working with independent professionals and all the cultural overtones that are inherent in that. For good or bad, the structure of general practice as it exists at present encompasses the two particular traits of independence and professionalism, and any comprehension of the way in which general practitioners function must be led by an understanding of what these traits signify.

General practices in the NHS have been independent contractors since its inception in 1948; general practitioners are self employed entrepreneurs who happen to contract with the NHS to provide primary care for patients of the NHS who register on their lists.

During the era of the FPC (and the Executive Councils before that) there was never a drive towards uniformity in the delivery of that provision. Over the years this led to a vast diversity in the range and standards of services provided, the types of premises, the number of doctors in a practice, and the size of list.

Seen in a positive sense, the variations in activity, which are often unexplained by demographic factors, have in recent years been an important part of the NHS "engine," driving progress onwards: motivated clinicians following their special interests and developing their own clinical "niches."

This idea of entrepreneurial pluralism leading to some (theoretical, at least) choice for patients is one that should clearly be encouraged, besides fitting in well with the current notions of a market driven health service. However, the negative side is that uncontrolled variation clearly poses a challenge in terms of maintaining and improving clinical standards.

Traditionally, the checks on such standards depended on an obligation to conform to nationally agreed requirements and the professionalism of the general practitioners. Part of the definition of any profession is its drive towards self improvement, and medicine has a long tradition of continuing education. As long as progress in medicine was predictable, and the expectations of general practice relatively low, self determined continuing education probably provided enough of a drive to maintain standards.

But times have changed, and so have public expectations of general practice and of the professions in general. Whether in the legal or medical professions, external legitimacy is now often sought, together with guarantees of minimum standards; neither of these fits in with the traditional concepts of professionalism, and this change needs to be taken into account in the planning of the management of general practice.

Several factors emerged as important in the development of general practice management in the 1990s:

- The necessity to plan the use of limited resources
- The requirement to maintain and improve standards
- The advantages of the independent contractor status
- The need to capitalise on professionalism in the context of heightened expectations.

The publication of the Government's White Paper *Working for patients*[1] was largely driven by the first two of these factors, and was instrumental in introducing the idea that general practice could be externally managed. What was less clear was the manner in which such management could be carried out.

The paper highlighted the necessity for accountability and responsiveness to the needs of a population. Although the notion of the independent contractor status of general practitioners was preserved, there was apparently no understanding of *why* such autonomy might be important, or why it might be useful to develop general practitioners' professionalism rather than undermining it. Regulation and constraint seemed to be the order of the day.

The one chink in this armour of restrictive management seemed to be medical audit: this was recognised as being an important discipline for general practitioners. It was to be a "professionally led, educational activity"[1] linked to management by an audit advisory group. Organised medical audit had arrived.

As has been illustrated in other chapters, professional audit has always been part of the medical culture; if it is part of the professional ethos to encourage self improvement, then it is clearly important to identify the areas where improvement is needed, which is precisely what medical audit is all about.

Among motivated doctors, informal self audit has always gone on, with practitioners learning from their experiences and their mistakes; the hospital consultant "*mea culpa*" sessions are well known both to medical students and to *aficionados* of the indulgent self flagellation school of education. Clinical audit projects are part of vocational training, and general practitioner practice meetings will often turn to ways of remedying perceived deficits in a service. It is often a very informal process, however, and one that does not always include all general practitioners. The challenge has been to discover how to involve those doctors who are not keen to carry out constructive critiques of their work.

Peer review, as suggested in the Royal College of General Practitioners' (RCGP's) "What sort of doctor" initiative,[2] has been seen as one way of encouraging audit in a manner that is much less threatening than review by any external body. Throughout the last years of the 1980s, however, the notion was implicit that, if the profession failed to get its own act together, then the bogey man of organisational audit would appear: "in the extreme case, those making the judgements may use the mechanism to control the status, income, or job security of doctor, nurse or group."[3]

Such a view, expressed by Marinker as recently as 1986, now seems at odds with the new "management culture" that pervades the NHS. Short term contracts and performance related pay are an integral part of a manager's working life, and managers do need effective levers to influence change, although such levers do not fit easily into the traditional patterns of medical care.

A medical carer needing to cope with the uncertainties of illness and prognosis requires a "safe" clinical environment, one that is stable and secure. For FHSAs to succeed in managing professionals effectively requires them to balance the need to improve standards of care at the trailing edge of general practice with the awareness that external control can destroy the safety and autonomy that good clinical practice requires.

Medical Audit Advisory Groups

The vehicle by which each FHSA was to promote audit, and encourage general practitioners to carry out assessments of their own work, was the Medical Audit Advisory Group (MAAG), a quasi-autonomous agency accountable to the FHSA, whose explicit target was the "participation of all practices [in medical audit] by April 1992."[4] Although the working paper "Medical audit and the family practitioner services" was relatively specific in its guidance about the membership and responsibilities of the MAAGs, FHSAs have interpreted this in a variety of ways, which have reflected the different purposes to which they have set MAAGs working.

In some instances (Baker R, personal communication), FHSAs have been very literal in their interpretation, insisting on the involvement of senior managers on the MAAG and, in one instance, even on the presence of a legal representative on the group. Other FHSAs have been much more relaxed about the constitution of the MAAG, and have taken a much more *laissez faire* attitude. The stance has depended very much on the *real* expectations made of the MAAGs, and these may be worth exploring further.

It has already been mentioned that, although self audit may be a laudable way of improving one's own performance, a certain degree of motivation is required to carry out such work. The first task of MAAGs was therefore to change the environment in which audit was perceived, and turn it into a tool for motivating and encouraging general practitioners.

The "new contract"[1] made an enormous impact on the way in which general practitioners worked, and on the way in which they perceived themselves and the organisation of the NHS. In spite of the fact that they had maintained their status as independent contractors, most general practitioners felt that their freedom of action had been largely if not wholly curtailed, and that the "new NHS" was a euphemism for a restrictive, punitive, line management system.

Any initiative that came from "the managers" was viewed with great cynicism and the suspicion that confrontation and control were the issues set to replace any idealism about patient care. Audit came burdened with financial and value laden overtones, both of which were guaranteed to present the very threat to which Marinker referred. To expect even the most progressive general practitioner to embrace this vision of medical audit was unreasonable, and so the more enlightened FHSAs set out initially to change the view that general practitioners had of audit, and of the FHSA itself.

They endeavoured to regain the status of the practitioners' friend, an organisation whose role was to help practices become more effective, and improve the services that they offered their patients. This status had been severely dented since 1990, and the new confrontational arrangements were leading to a loss of enthusiasm and a retraction among some general practitioners into a demotivated "Jobsworth" mentality. Entrepreneurialism was being stifled, and the whole *raison d'être* of the independent contractor status was at risk.

So how could the MAAGs be constituted in such a way that FHSA/general practitioner relations would be improved?

Firstly, most MAAGs were funded and managed in a very "hands off" manner. The selection of members was in many cases left to the local professionals to determine; the regulations stipulated that there be representation from the Local Medical Committee, the local faculty of the RCGP, an academic input from a university department of general practice, and a public health medicine presence. In addition, a balance of different groups of general practitioners, such as those from large and small practices, fundholders and non-fundholders, urban and rural, as well as an ethnic and gender mix, was selected by the FHSA. The progressive early MAAGs felt very much like talking shops for general practitioners.

Secondly, in many of the early MAAGs, formal FHSA representation was not apparent and so there were no obvious external drivers to the agenda. The General Medical Services Committee (GMSC) issued guidance which suggested that even the independent medical adviser, as an employee of the FHSA, should be excluded from the MAAG,[5] and certainly it was rare to find an "administrator" on the MAAG. The presence of a legal representative on one MAAG was sufficiently exceptional to get wide media coverage, and his fate is not recorded. Suffice it to say that it went against the grain of the style of the early MAAGs.

153

Thirdly, and most importantly, some MAAGs saw that their initial task was more about consciousness raising than about the carrying out of particularly important clinical audits. If the body of general practioners was to be persuaded to carry out medical audit of its own accord then its apprehensions and cynical misgivings would have to be defused.

The manner in which members of individual MAAGs carried out their tasks varied in different FHSA areas; some saw themselves as "executives," whose role was to set a strategic direction for local audit activities and to delegate the operational work to audit facilitators (for example, Leicestershire[6]). Others saw themselves in the role of those facilitators, visiting practices, discussing projects, and acting as an information resource for individual doctors (for example, North Tyneside[7]). Somewhere in between these two there were other MAAGs, whose members carried out selective visits, exhorting the troops, and disseminating encouragement and good ideas (for example, Devon[8]).

Given that the key task in the early days was the raising of general practitioners' audit awareness, the actual audit subjects were seen as relatively unimportant. Outcome audits are always difficult to carry out in primary care, where it is not easy to make a causal connection between activity and outcome (usually because we do not really know what outcome we should be looking at!), and hence much of the work looked at procedural audit or, when even that was difficult, at structural audit.

Thus, work was carried out evaluating the "how" of practice, with very little of the "what." For instance, the Leicestershire vitamin B_{12} study (Fraser RC, personal communication) encouraged practices to follow the classic audit cycle pathway. General practitioners started by establishing the desired patterns of vitamin B_{12} usage among their patients and devising a method by which their own activity in the field could be measured. They then implemented a change policy if their activity was at odds with these criteria, and revisited the study at a later date to see whether change had occurred and been sustained.

Many of them started the study with the perception that their own activity was exemplary, and were horrified to discover that this was not the case at all! The resulting "startle factor" was often a great stimulus to further work in the project, and a general irritant to clinical complacency in other fields. The project thus achieved several aims:

- The use of vitamin B_{12} was rationalised and clinical practice improved
- Complacency was disturbed and curiosity aroused
- Audit methodology was learned and used
- The perceptual difficulties of medical audit were defused
- The threat of audit was considerably reduced
- The image of the MAAG as a support was strengthened.

At the start of the project, over 80% of practitioners were committed to it, and it is interesting to compare this figure with South Glamorgan,[10] where only 44% of practices were involved in a similar district wide audit of diabetes. The clinical significance of such a project is clearly greater, which makes it more important from the point of view of health gain, but its very significance is bound to make the threat of the audit much greater, and hence perhaps less suitable as an educational introduction to medical audit.

In some cases, even a process audit may have been seen as threatening, or too difficult, and then it may have been considering carrying out a structural audit.

Such audits really lie in the grey zone between medical audit and organisational audit, *à la* King's Fund or the British Standards Institute. Clinicians are likely to feel less threatened (and, of course, less involved) if they are asked to audit their appointment system than if they are expected to test out their standards of clinical care. For educational purposes, the methodology is the same, but the appointment system is less likely to provoke curiosity and self motivation than standards of clinical care. Pragmatism suggests that process audit, as the middle path, is the most likely to be powerful enough to drive change without being so intrusive as to provoke rejection.

Effectiveness of clinical audit

One of the problems that underlay this approach to MAAGs was that its own effectiveness was difficult to measure. The Department of Health was concerned with promoting changes in clinical behaviour (MAAGs should "ensure changes in professional practice when these are required"[4]), albeit through the development of strategies for local audit. Public money to the tune of £5–10 million was being protected for medical audit in primary care on a recurring basis, and accountability was being sought.

There was a feeling outside that, inside the Department of Health, there was an ongoing tension between those who were prepared to let MAAGs fulfil this "change agency" role and those who wanted to see concrete, measurable outcomes to medical audit occurring from the start. For the first three years, the first group have had their way, and FHSAs have been content to continue funding MAAGs on the basis of the process in which they were engaged.

The "change agency" lobby have, however, only managed to maintain this position by arguing that the "product," when it finally arrived, would be worth the wait and, by so doing, have raised the expectations of what that product might actually be. It must have clinical significance, it must encompass diseases that are common, and it should try to marry the medical and management agendas together.

To do this, medical audit is gradually maturing to include the management view. Increasingly, MAAGs are starting to engage their FHSAs directly, and are beginning to discuss potential areas of audit that meet the needs of both groups. The NHS Executive needs FHSAs to show that change is occurring and that the MAAG money is not being wasted, and MAAGs themselves are realising that their survival depends on producing results. So the defensive "hands off our MAAG" view is changing as MAAGs and FHSAs begin to collaborate, and to produce outputs that have external legitimacy.

Disease areas such as diabetes and asthma are being audited, and protocols based on the results are appearing. Moreover, other innovations are being made that help to strengthen the relevance of the audit process. One of these is the move from medical audit towards clinical audit.

Clinical audit versus medical audit

The "traditional" MAAG was wholly medical in its outlook; it may have employed facilitators from other disciplines, but the thinking and philosophy were very much in the medical mould. Clinical audit, on the other hand, acknowledges the fact that if the impact of health care is to be measured effectively, then a more holistic view of that care needs to be taken. It is not just the general practitioner's bedside manner or prescribing that affects clinical care and its outcomes, but also the training and clinical behaviour of the nurse, the telephone manners of the receptionist, and the advice given by the pharmacist. Clinical audit should be able to encompass all these, and more, so that the emerging standards and changes in behaviour will be more likely to improve the whole standard of care.

To this end, many MAAGs now include paramedical staff among their numbers, primarily nurses, but potentially all the other staff (including managers??) who are involved in the provision of health care. In the same way as clinical audit needs to encompass many allied disciplines, so it must cross other traditional boundaries.

So far, most MAAGs have carried out all their work in the boundaries set by general practice. Cross boundary audit is, however, slowly beginning to appear, allowing care to be measured and improved in a much broader sphere. The most significant aspect of cross sectoral audit is that of the primary/secondary care interface.

Audit across the primary/secondary care interface

In the same way that medical audit is not complete because it excludes all the other "players" in health care, so single sector audit is dramatically incomplete because it does not consider all the variables that may affect the outcome of an intervention. Thus, asthma care within the primary care sector may exclude the impact of hospital admissions, outpatient attendances, retail pharmacists' advice, or information from the British Thoracic Society. It is clearly pointless to effect change in practice which impinges on these other sectors without understanding what the consequences on these sectors are likely to be.

Similarly, hospital audit activities tend to stop at the point of patient discharge, and there are certainly no formal mechanisms for carrying out audits between hospitals and general practices. Postoperative discharges are being made earlier and earlier, and the only way in which they impact on the community services tends to be measured in readmission rates, or the number of outpatient follow up visits. The sooner MAAG activities are coordinated with hospital audits, the sooner it will be possible to measure the genuine and complete effects of medical interventions.

The same could be said about other interfaces, such as those between medicine and social services, medicine and social security, medicine and education, and even medicine and housing, but such ideas may still be a little radical for the time being.

Clinical audit in benchmark setting

Once the notion of cross sectoral audit has been introduced, it leaves the way open for the development of cross sectoral audit standards, and the setting of clinical benchmarks. Such ideas tie together several of the themes that have already been discussed.

The process is led by clinicians, without the threat of managerial overbearance, and so participating doctors feel an ownership of the process and its results. It has a genuine use, with a potential impact on significant parts of the health care system. It ties in with managerial imperatives to coordinate the delivery of services, and to ensure efficiency and cost effectiveness. It provides a template for cross sectoral working, producing "shared care guidelines" of the best sort. Its results become *de facto* minimum standards which are then difficult for clinicians to disregard.

Once the concept of minimum clinical standards has been accepted on this positive basis, then the idea of working towards such minimum standards will inevitably be raised. Can audit be used to ensure minimum standards? Is it reasonable to expect new doctors to be accredited in specified clinical areas before they are allowed to practise in those areas? Should it actually be doctors who are accredited, or multidisciplinary teams? And what about existing practitioners who are not maintaining such standards; should they be identified? If they are identified, what should happen to them? What is the place of audit in *re*accreditation, whether in a remedial sense or in the sense of continuing professional education?

If these questions were to be raised in a managerial environment, clinicians would quite rightly resent and fear them. In the context of professionally driven clinical audit, however, there is no reason why all these notions should not be accepted and even welcomed. If audit is to have an effect on working practices and standards, it would be foolish not to incorporate these into everyday "norms" in some way. The clinicians who have identified the standards and worked to achieve them would not be pleased if other less motivated teams did not bother to attempt the same tasks.

Professional pride should drive all those concerned in providing patient care to improve their performance, and audit of this type seems an ideal way of developing that professionalism. If new doctors wish to join this professional "élite," then it seems reasonable for them to establish their clinical credentials before starting to practise. Even the suggestion that it should be teams rather than individuals who are accredited in a particular clinical area is not as outlandish as it first sounds. It capitalises on the fact that good audit crosses sectoral boundaries, and acknowledges that in a team each member is valued for his or her individual contribution to the whole.

It also makes sense for those who have difficulty keeping up with the standard (which would itself be changing and rising with each turn of the audit cycle) to be helped. Once again, it is the professional aspects of clinical audit that make it useful in these circumstances. If the process were managerially driven, then the prevailing perception (if not the reality) would be of sanctions and penalties. Through ownership by the clinicians, reaccreditation becomes an issue of catching up and rethinking, welcomed by those who need it, and perceived in a negative way only by those who refuse to take part in the process.

The practical reality is that a nationally agreed contract for "general medical services" is rapidly becoming unworkable.

The move of care out of institutions into the community means that workloads in primary care are rising, without any professional or financial recognition. If the move is to continue, then the implications must be considered. Quality will need to be assured, teams developed to deliver the care, and the practical quantification of the work will be required to attribute resources (in the widest sense) to that care. Where primary care teams are providing some care themselves, and purchasing the rest from secondary providers, then clarity of workload, its quality, and its effectiveness are vital pieces of the care jigsaw.

Thus, in many parts of the country, general practitioners are beginning to accept that local contracting for primary care may not be far off. Some are positively welcoming the notion, because it means that they can extend the range and quality of their services, knowing that these will be acceptable to patients, to purchasers, and to their own high clinical standards. In the context of a primary care focused health care system, paying practices for the work that they are actually prepared to do, at a standard that is guaranteed, must be the cornerstone of progress, and is probably not practicable within the mechanisms of the existing national contract.

The management perspective

Finally, it may be worth looking at the whole concept of clinical audit from a slightly different viewpoint. This chapter has so far considered the advantages of autonomous, professionally driven audit as a tool for improving clinical standards, and for facilitating communications between clinical professional groups, as well as between clinicians and managers. Considering it as an organisational tool for the growth and development of clinical care allows us to consider audit from the management perspective.

Since 1990 the structure of the NHS has been split between those who commission and purchase care (DHAs and FHSAs) and those who provide it (in primary care and in hospitals).

As time passes, however, it is becoming clearer that the commissioners of care have the extra responsibility of ensuring that their local providers can deliver appropriate care to the requisite standards of quality and quantity. In particular, the range and quality of the services provided by general practices are enormously variable; the independent nature of this sector, and the small size of its organisations, also mean that it will never be in a position to develop the necessary quality markers entirely on its own. In addition, general practice providers are extending their role from that of provider alone to being commissioner as well, and this learning curve is a steep one indeed.

Professionally led clinical audit, facilitated and funded by the commissioning agencies, provides the ideal tool with which to manage this conundrum. We have seen how it can encourage the development of motivation, self direction, and professional self esteem. It can have an impressive effect on clinical standards and, if it is multidisciplinary, the working practices that result can be applied across different sectors. The standards that emerge can become the benchmarks against which clinicians can measure themselves, and against which new practitioners may be assessed. It provides a means for general practices to measure the effectiveness of *their* providers (that is, hospitals) and so help them to purchase secondary care appropriately.

And finally, but most importantly, professionally led clinical audit remains within the control of its participants; it is the ideal tool for measuring and changing clinical practice, attitudes, and interprofessional relationships.

1 *Working for patients.* Secretaries of State for Social Services for England, Wales, Northern Ireland and Scotland. London: HMSO, 1989. Cm249.
2 *What sort of doctor?*: Report from General Practice 23. London: Royal College of General Practitioners, 1985.
3 Marinker M, Performance review and professional values. In: Pendleton DA, Schofield TPC, Marinker M, eds, *Pursuit of quality.* London: RCGP, 1986.
4 Working for Patients, Health Service Development. *Medical audit in the family practitioner services.* Department of Health Circular HC (FP) (90) 8, 1990.
5 *GMSC Annual Report.* Appendix XVIII. London: GMSC, 1991.
6 Sorrie R, Darling L. Leicestershire MAAG report. *Audit Trends* 1993; 1(1):28–9.
7 Southern A. North Tyneside MAAG report. *Audit Trends* 1993; 1(2): 73–4.
8 Stead J. Devon MAAG report. *Audit Trends* 1993; 1(2):68.
9 Voisey J. South Glamorgan MAAG report. *Audit Trends* 1993; 1(4): 175–6.

10 Audit in fundholding: evaluating purchasing performance

BRIAN M GOSS

The General Practitioner Fundholding Scheme which began in 1990 marked a new phase in relationships between general practitioners and other professional colleagues. By placing the purchase of certain types of NHS services under the direct control of referring general practitioners, the power of secondary and community care providers to determine priorities in resource allocation was severely curtailed. This change required delicate adjustments in traditional patterns of interchange, particularly between general practitioners and consultant colleagues.

That delicacy has to be carried into any understanding of the role of audit when it applies to the work of other professionals, be they hospital doctors, community staff, or physiotherapists. It is an important principle of audit that it should be an agreed activity undertaken by peers who themselves determine the performance criteria against which they should be measured.

In assessing their work as purchasers, general practitioner fundholders (and, of equal importance, other purchasers) must be sensitive to the fact that they must not interfere with the audit processes of the professionals within the provider units themselves.

The resources available for auditing performance are limited to what is left of the Practice Fund Management Allowance (PFMA) after the required accounting functions have been undertaken and the necessary reports produced. This chapter is not intended to represent any minimum standard for fundholding audit, but rather to explore possible avenues of self assessment which are open to practices as their purchasing sophistication develops.

How then can purchasing audit be constructed? The first requirement of audit is the agreement of a standard. In the context of fundholding, the appropriate places for the expression of standards are the purchasing plan and the service agreements, which should be written with an intrinsic capability to form the standard against which purchasing performance can be assessed.

There are two main ways in which purchasers can influence the quality of care delivered: choice of provider and contract monitoring.

Choice of provider

In the early days of fundholding, the stability of the traditional NHS providers was a major consideration. Increasingly, other factors are able to influence the setting of contracts. For the first few years, access times have been an issue of key importance. Published figures of outpatient and inpatient waiting times are able to inform purchasing intentions. More recently the aggregated waiting time from referral to procedure (what I like to call the "pen to knife" time) has become more readily available.

Some providers are producing more sophisticated quality information, including outcome measures and infection rates on procedures. Where truly comparable data are available, allowing purchasers to make comparisons that take account of the effects of case mix (units taking "difficult" cases are likely to have "worse" outcomes), such data can inform a rational choice of provider.

Other aspects of quality are increasingly being built into contracts. The grade of staff seen in hospitals, the grade of nurse undertaking various parts of the community nursing function, and the steps taken to inform patients of the clinical procedures proposed are possible areas for finding measurable proxies for quality.

In terms of patient convenience, the failure to provide necessary drugs and certification at discharge or in outpatients is a potent source of irritation, which can be addressed through the contracting process. Increasingly contractual penalties are being put in place where these basic services are not rendered.

The audit standards which can properly be set by fundholders as purchasers in assessing their choice of providers therefore include:

- Providers being chosen on the basis of published information which addresses access times for consultations and procedures
- The referral to procedure time
- The case mix controlled outcome
- The grade of staff dealing with patients.

Contracts should enforce patient convenience issues such as the provision of drugs and the provision of certification. These criteria should be referred to in the purchasing plan, and be enforceable through the service agreements.

Contract monitoring

Although the Practice Fund Management Allowance is thought to be generous by the detractors of fundholding, the large amount of keyboard inputting time required by the accounting system leaves little resource for the mechanics of data retrieval and manipulation which are required for audit. Ideally the fundholding software itself should be set up to provide as much of the audit data as possible, leaving a minimal amount to be monitored using external spreadsheets, involving inevitable duplicate entry of data. Although the much criticised, fundholding, software specification does not readily lend itself to contract monitoring or clinical audit, the implementation of certain procedural rules can enable standard reports to be adapted for audit purposes. The referral exception report (Fund report 2) is the most useful in this respect. This report identified activities that have not been "commenced" by the "expected date," so that careful attention to the setting of the expected date greatly enhances the usefulness of the report.

Access and waiting times are particular examples. Having negotiated particular access times with provider units, the expected interval between referral and activity can be set for each procedure code in each unit. These become the default expected date when each referral is logged on to the system. Where clinical priority dictates an earlier date, the expected date can be modified on an individual basis.

An extension of this manipulation can be applied to the monitoring of pen to knife times for elective surgery when the referring general practitioner has a clear idea of the required procedure. If, at the time of initial referral, a fundholding referral note is generated in respect of the probable procedure, as well as the outpatient consultation, the expected date should be entered to reflect the contracted or desired time from initial referral to performance of the procedure.

If both these procedures are followed, referral exception reports can be generated for each provider unit showing the procedures at regular intervals. A detailed listing can be extracted so that the patients who have been referred to hospital A for cataract removal, but have not been operated on within six months of referral, can be readily identified. This allows not only for audit, but for action in terms of contract enforcement or alternative referral to be undertaken in time for purchasing objectives to be met.

It is important to recognise that the expected times must reflect reality, otherwise referral exception reports become massive and unwieldy—they should be short and target cases where effective action can be taken. It is perhaps best to think of the expected date in the same terms as a bring forward file, so that any patient appearing on a referral exception report truly does merit clinical or management action. This is particularly true of outpatient attendances where, because of the sheer numbers involved, reports can very easily grow to unmanageable proportions.

Monitoring of other more direct quality aspects of care requires other methods which are not within the fundholding software. The two principal methods are reporting of breaches by general practitioners and the establishment of patient satisfaction questionnaires. These questionnaires are highly labour intensive in terms of analysis and require careful targeting on known problem areas.

In non-fundholding practices, similar purchasing audit can be done on behalf of the purchasing authority. Where waiting lists are provided by hospitals this is made much simpler, although the information still needs to be fed onto spreadsheets for verification and analysis. The resources for audit, of course, have to come from a different source in the absence of a management allowance.

Whether in a fundholding or non-fundholding environment, purchasing audit needs to be targeted at known problem areas if best use is to be made of audit resources and for the best chance of obtaining information that will be effective in delivering enhanced patient care.

11 Statistical issues in medical audit

DAPHNE RUSSELL, IAN RUSSELL

In this chapter, we show how statistical principles can help in the conduct and then the interpretation of an audit. To set this discussion in context we first identify some of the differences and similarities between medical audit and medical research—the activity within medicine with which the application of statistical principles is traditionally associated.

Audit and research: differences and similarities

Most statistical advice to doctors in lectures and textbooks is directed towards the doctor doing research. Much of this also applies to audit, but there are at least three important differences.

First, the researcher, even if the data come from only a few practices (or even one!), is interested in drawing inferences about a general population of patients, doctors, or practices; he or she will usually concentrate on a small subset of practice activities. In contrast, an audit seeks to draw inferences about only one doctor or practice, but will aim (eventually) to cover a representative selection of practice activities.

Second, in audit a given practice's results are compared with a predetermined standard so that the appropriate statistical procedure is a hypothesis test answering the question "Are we falling significantly short of the standard?" Although hypothesis tests are used in research, the researcher is more often interested in estimation—for example, by confidence intervals.

Third, most researchers either compare two or more samples or investigate the relationship between many variables. In audit a

166

single sample is compared with a standard, one variable at a time.

In spite of these differences, the doctor undertaking audit needs to abide by most of the basic principles of research: precision in defining objectives and procedures; careful planning so that the data he or she needs are available, unbiased, and reliable; rigorous sampling methods and statistical analysis; and clear presentation of results and conclusions.

Sampling and bias

Enumerate or sample?

When comparing practice performance with a specified standard one may either enumerate all relevant patients within the practice or sample only some of the relevant patients and infer from them the overall practice performance.

Enumeration should be used where the standard of interest refers to routine and readily available statistics, often already compiled for another purpose. Examples in chapter 13 include causes of death (table 13.2, page 206) and major diagnoses (table 13.3, page 206). Even when numbers are large and sampling would give adequate estimates, it is as easy (or easier) to count all patients, provided that the data needed are already in the practice computer. As the information held on practice computers becomes more sophisticated and detailed, the range of topics for which enumeration is feasible will increase. Enumeration will also be necessary if the event of interest is so rare that all relevant patients need to be examined.

Example 1—In any one year there will be relatively few cancer deaths in a single practice (see, for example, table 13.2, page 206). If you want to compare your terminal care with an agreed protocol you should use all such patients even if extra work is required for the comparison.

Sampling is recommended, however, whenever a detailed analysis of the whole practice or a large subgroup of patients, consultations, or activities is required. Limiting audit to areas that can be enumerated easily is too restrictive.

The detailed analysis may be done retrospectively by examining existing records or prospectively by using an extra recording sheet for the sampled patients or consultations to provide more detail than would otherwise be available. An example of retrospective analysis is given in table 13.5 (page 207), in which patients' records of 160 patients sampled from over 5000 were examined for information on smoking. As an example of an ambitious prospective audit one might sample 10% of hospital referrals and seek additional information from the referring doctor during the initiating consultation, the hospital consultant during the first outpatient visit, and the patient by post after discharge from the outpatient clinic.

The first step in sampling is to define the population—the entire set of items or measurements of interest.[1] To audit the treatment within a practice of a chronic disease such as asthma or diabetes, for example, one might define the population as all patients in the practice with the specified condition. For an acute illness such as childhood vomiting, however, a more appropriate population may be patients who consult the doctor about that illness within a given period. A sample is any subset of the population of interest that is used to draw conclusions about that population.

Example 2—Fifty of the hospital referrals from the practice in a given year could be examined in detail by drawing one of the following samples (of which only the last is at all representative):

- The first 50 referrals in the year of interest
- Half the patients referred by the trainee
- All the medical and geriatric referrals
- The first referral in each of 50 weeks in the year.

The process of drawing conclusions about a population from a sample is called statistical inference. The quality of the inference depends on both the sample size and how representative of the population the sample is.

Bias occurs when the sample is not representative of the population. It may occur at either or both of two stages: the definition of the sampling frame—a list of all the members of the population; and the choice of sampling procedure—the way in which items are selected from the sampling frame.

Sampling frames

The best sampling frame contains one and only one entry for each member of the population of interest. Most sampling frames, however, suffer from one or more of the following defects:

- Missing elements, which should be listed but are not
- Foreign elements, which should not be listed but are
- Duplicated elements, that is, many entries for one element
- Clustered elements, that is, one entry for many elements.

Example 3—To sample from all episodes of illness in the practice you could use the appointments book as a sampling frame. This method would include all the defects above:

- Illnesses seen only by the practice nurse
- Patients who made appointments but did not attend
- Episodes of illness with two or more consultations
- Separate consultations for two or more family members within the same appointment.

Example 4—To sample from all patients referred to hospital during 1995 copies of referral letters could be used as a sampling frame. There would probably be missing elements (for example, emergency admissions), foreign elements (for example, temporary residents), and duplicated elements (for example, patients referred more than once during the year), but there would probably be no clustered elements unless one letter was used to refer two or more patients.

As far as possible such errors should be corrected or allowed for, otherwise the sampling frame will not be representative of the population.

Sampling procedure

The aim is to make the sample representative of the sampling frame. *Judgment samples* are personally selected, often using a quota system. But they are usually unrepresentative, and statistical inferences are rarely safe. Therefore some form of *random sampling* will almost always be necessary; every item on the sampling frame should have a chance of being selected.

In a *simple random sample* every possible sample, and therefore every item, has an equal chance of being selected. Fully computerised records are the easiest to sample; with one or two commands or options you should be able to produce a computer file containing a specified number or a specified percentage of the original records. Otherwise you will need to allocate a number to each item in the sampling frame, and use a list of *random numbers* to choose those items whose numbers appear in this list. As random numbers are equally likely to take any value, the items in the sampling frame may be numbered in any convenient way—for example, alphabetical or chronological. Sorting the chosen random numbers from smallest to largest (often possible by computer) will quickly show which should be discarded and, if numbers have been allocated in sequence, make it easier to extract the relevant data.

Example 5—To choose 20 out of 880 consultations for a given "tracer condition", generate a list of 20 three digit random numbers (equally likely to take any value between 000 and 999), discard and replace any that are larger than 880 or repeat a number already in the list, and use those consultations whose numbers appear in the final list. All computers, and many hand calculators, can generate random numbers with a given number of digits. If no computer is available, you should use a random number table (for example, that on page 9 of Bland[2]).

Sometimes it may be easier to use a *systematic sample*: in Example 5, for instance, one could use a single random number to choose one of the first 44 consultations, and thereafter take every 44th. Every sample item is equally likely to be chosen as each belongs to precisely one of the 44 possible samples. There is, however, a risk of bias if, say, there are about 22 relevant consultations a week and Monday consultations differ from Friday consultations.

Sample size

An unbiased sample chosen by a good sampling procedure from a good sampling frame will give estimates that have no systematic tendency to be too large or too small. An individual estimate from a single sample may, however, diverge substantially from the *parameter* to be estimated (the true underlying value), especially if the sample is too small. Too small a sample will fail to label as significantly below the predetermined standard any performance that falls so far below that standard as to be clinically important. Too large a sample, as well as wasting effort, will label as significantly below standard a performance that is nevertheless close enough for the difference to be of no clinical importance.

170

Example 6—Suppose that the desired standard for the immunisation rate among two year olds in the practice is 90%, that a shortfall of 10% is considered clinically important, and that you would like to detect such a shortfall from the standard on at least 95% of the occasions on which it occurs. Then statistical calculations along the lines described by Bland[2] can be used to calculate the sample size needed: in this example it is about 133 children.

Note that this example could be interpreted as a criticism of a key element of the general practitioner contract, which takes no account of practice size when awarding target payments. A rate of only 85% in a small practice could be a random fluctuation from a "satisfactory" performance and a rate of 90% could be a random fluctuation from an "unsatisfactory" performance. Even worse, the clinically insignificant difference between 89% and 90% may be most significant financially.

Validity and reliability

As well as avoiding bias in the sample it is important to ensure that one is measuring what one wants to measure. It is desirable to check on this both in planning the audit and on a subsample of the patients whose care is being audited.

Example 7—Blood pressure measurements vary according to the attitude of the patient (standing, sitting, or lying), the interval since exercise, and the identity of the measurer (doctor, nurse, or patient).[3] The diagnosis of asthma varies substantially between general practitioners.[4] When auditing the care of chronic conditions such as hypertension and asthma you should therefore use well defined diagnostic criteria.

Reliability measures internal consistency: if the measurement is repeated under the same conditions how much will it vary?

Example 8—In Example 7 repeated blood pressure measurements by the same measurer on the same patient in the same attitude will provide a measure of reliability.

Validity measures consistency with the "gold standard." Is the measurement correct? If not, how well does it correlate with the gold standard?

Example 9—Even if the gold standard for blood pressure is based on measurement when the patient is lying down, measurement when the patient is standing can be used for audit if its bias is more or less consistent—for example, between 10% and 20% above the lying measurement—but not if it is sometimes 20% below and sometimes 20% above.

Checking reliability

This is an important component of audit—often more important than checking validity. The methods available include the following:

1 Repeated measurement, for example, of blood pressure. This is not always possible, however. For instance, the reliability of a questionnaire on patients' knowledge of asthma cannot usefully be tested by sending second copies of the questionnaire to the same patients, because this is likely merely to test their memories of their previous answers.
2 Measurement by another partner or member of the primary care team, for example, to assess the accuracy with which an outcome like hearing loss has been measured.
3 Measurement by another method, such as a postal questionnaire to the patient or a self administered blood sugar reading.

Of these methods the first is likely to show the smallest variation. But it may not be superior to the other methods if it causes too much reliance to be placed on a measurement whose value is highly dependent on who is doing the measuring. If Dr A always measures blood pressure when the patient is standing, and Dr B always measures it when the patient is lying down, knowledge of the measurement alone is not an adequate guide to whether a patient should be classified as hypertensive.

Checking validity

Although the gold standard is sometimes available in general practice, checking validity will more often entail direct comparison with hospital or laboratory data.

172

Analysing the data

The purpose of analysing the data from a practice audit is to compare results from that practice with a fixed standard so as to answer the question "Is the practice meeting the standard for this activity?" There may also be a subsidiary question: "By how much do we fall short of the standard?"

If only a sample of the relevant patients is used, *statistical analysis* is needed to draw inferences about the population from the sample. Even if all relevant patients are used, statistical analysis will still be appropriate if these patients represent a sample from the population of all patients who could have had the condition that is the subject of the audit. Inferences may be of three types, depending on the sample data:

1 There is significant evidence that practice performance is below the standard
2 There is significant evidence that practice performance is above the standard
3 There is insufficient evidence that practice performance differs from the standard.

The choice between (1), (2), and (3), or more realistically between (1) and (3), needs a *hypothesis test*. If an answer to the subsidiary question is also needed a *confidence interval* is appropriate.

Example 10—Suppose the practice has decided to aim for a standard that requires that 70% of adult male patients should have had their blood pressures recorded within the past five years. Suppose further that out of a sample of 100 only 60 records show such a reading. Can we infer that the practice is not meeting the standard?

If the practice is meeting the standard precisely then on average a sample of 100 men will include 70 "successes" (patients whose blood pressure has been recorded). We would not be at all surprised if there were 69 or 71 successes but we do expect the number of successes to be close to 70.

There are thus two possible explanations for the observed success rate of 60%:

(a) The practice is meeting the standard but an unlikely event has occurred: we have chosen a sample in which only 60 men have

173

their blood pressure recorded, rather than the 70 men that might have been expected.

(b) The practice is not meeting the standard; fewer than 70% of male patients in the practice have had their blood pressure recorded.

The usual statistical approach is to accept the first explanation unless the chance of the "unlikely event" is extremely small, typically less than 5%. If so, the second explanation is preferred to the first and conclusion (1) applies: the proportion of male patients whose blood pressure has been recorded is *significantly* below 70%. However, if the "unlikely event" is not so very unlikely, occurring in rather more than 5% of practices that are meeting this standard, conclusion (3) will apply: there is insufficient evidence to say the proportion of male patients whose blood pressure has been recorded is significantly below 70%.

Provided that the sample of 100 patients has been randomly chosen, we can use the mathematical theory of variation among repeated samples from the same population to calculate the chance of the "unlikely event" occurring (usually described as the *significance level*). This is one of the strongest arguments for using random samples; in a judgment sample, even if the bias is not large, there is no way of calculating how unlikely an atypical sample is.

The calculations can be done on many hand calculators. The method is given in most introductory medical statistics textbooks (for example, Bland[2]), and illustrated in the Appendix using Example 10 above. If, however, you have access to a statistical computer package (or a statistically minded colleague) and are happy to use either of these as a "black box," the number of people you sampled, the number who were dealt with correctly, and the proportion you would consider satisfactory will be used to calculate how likely you would be to get a sample as bad as the one you actually got, if the overall practice performance were satisfactory.

In Example 10, we find that the chance that a sample from a practice that is meeting the standard would have as few as 60 out of 100 successes is only 0·015 (1·5%). This chance is much less than the usual criterion of 5%. Thus rather than believing that such an unlikely event has occurred we prefer to conclude that the *proportion of male patients whose blood pressure has been recorded is significantly below 70%*. There is evidence (at the 5% level) that the practice is not meeting the standard (conclusion (1) on page 173).

What would have happened if we had sampled fewer than 100 patients? We could also have got a 60% "success rate" by using only 40 men in the sample and finding 24 "successes." Now the chance of getting a sample as bad as this from a practice exactly meeting the standard is 0·082 (8·2%). As this is larger than the usual criterion of 5%, we should conclude that the "unlikely event" is not sufficiently unlikely to reject the first explanation. A sample of this size might well estimate the success rate at 60% or below even if the practice were meeting the standard. So here we prefer the second explanation and conclude that *the proportion of male patients whose blood pressure has been recorded is not significantly different from 70%*. There is not enough evidence (at the 5% level) to state that the practice is not meeting the standard (conclusion (3) on page 173).

Note the difference between the two cases: although both samples have the same proportion of successes, this is judged to be significantly below the standard only in the first case, because the larger the sample size the less the population and sample are likely to differ.

Example 11—Example 6 suggested that a sample size of 133 was needed to compare a practice immunisation rate with an agreed standard of 90%. Provided that a sample of this size is achieved, calculations similar to those in the Appendix would establish that a sample immunisation rate of 85% or less was significantly below the desired standard of 90%. Sample rates lower than 85% are unlikely to occur when the practice as a whole is meeting the standard. A sample rate between 86% and 90% is not, however, sufficiently unlikely in a practice that is meeting the standard to justify the conclusion that this practice as a whole is not meeting the standard.

If the practice genuinely has an "unsatisfactory" rate of only 80% this will be detected unless the sample happens to have an immunisation rate above 85%—higher than the overall practice rate. The sample size of 133 has been chosen so that 95% of samples from such a practice will have rates of 85% or lower and thus lead to the correct conclusion that performance is

175

unsatisfactory, even though the remaining 5% of samples would lead to an incorrect conclusion.

Confidence intervals for Example 10

The best estimate for the true rate of blood pressure recording in that practice is 60/100 (60%). Many other true population percentages could, however, have given rise to the sample that we have observed. If the sample is not biased the most likely population percentages are close to 60% and the least likely are much larger or smaller than 60%.

A *confidence interval*[5] gives a range of population percentages which is likely (usually 95% or 99% likely) to include the true one. The Appendix shows that a 95% confidence interval for the true rate of blood pressure recording in the practice of Example 10 lies between 50·4% and 69·6%. A 99% confidence interval lies between 47·5% and 72·5%. Although the second interval is wider it is more likely to include the true rate.

Types of test

Example 10 uses a test of a single proportion from a "large" sample. Different tests arise from different types of data and sizes of sample. For other tests and the conditions under which they are valid one should consult an introductory medical statistics textbook (for example, Bland[2]). Conclusions usually take the form of a confidence interval[5] for a practice percentage, average, or other parameter of interest, and a statement about practice performance similar to (1), (2), or (3) on page 173, qualified by the relevant significance level.

Note that statement (3) does not imply that the standard is being met, merely that the evidence is not strong enough to say that it is not being met. If the confidence interval is very wide the sample size is probably too small. The best remedy is to take a larger sample, preferably of the size suggested by calculations similar to those reported in Example 6.

Presenting the audit

Target audience

You will gain more from your audit if results are summarised in tables or graphs and conclusions are clearly stated. In addition, you will often wish to present your findings to colleagues within the practice, for example, when suggesting changes. You may also wish to send a report to the local Medical Audit Advisory Group (or the equivalent in Scotland or Northern Ireland).

Structure of report

The traditional structure for medical publications provides a useful basis for an audit report:

1 Summary—a few hundred words to tell the reader:
   (a) which standard you adopted
   (b) how your performance compared with it
   (c) how you propose to bring your performance closer to your standard (revised if necessary).
2 Introduction, with particular reference to:
   (a) which topic you chose and why
   (b) which standard you adopted and why.
3 Method, covering at least five basic components:
   (a) basic design (what you did in general terms)
   (b) sampling (how?)
   (c) data collection (how?)
   (d) data validation (how you checked your data and with what result)
   (e) analysis (how you compared your performance with the standard).
4 Results, using tables or graphs where appropriate.
5 Discussion, critically appraising both your audit method and your performance.
6 Conclusions and recommendations, in particular:
   (a) whether your standard should now be revised
   (b) how you propose to bring your performance closer to it.

The case for tables

Tables are the basic tool for presenting your results; several examples are given in chapter 13. They provide an effective way of summarising a set of figures. As an example compare the following paragraph with table 11.1 (both derived from table 13.4, page 206):

In 1994 Dr DAH had 1274 patients under 65, 213 aged between 65 and 74, and 205 older patients; Dr MAP had 991 patients aged 64 or less, 178 aged between 65 and 74, and 154 aged 75 or older; Dr PJD had 1597 patients under 65, 180 aged between 65 and 74, and 132 aged 75 or older; and Dr AGD had 564 patients under 65, 54 between 65 and 74, and 28 aged over 75.

Table 11.1

Age group	Doctor			
	DAH	MAP	PJD	AGD
64 or less	1274	991	1597	564
65–74	213	178	180	54
75 or more	205	154	132	28

Even this table can be improved as the following guidelines for tables suggest.

How to present tables

1 Give the table a title that is helpful and clear but as concise as possible; label rows and columns even more concisely.
2 It is usually best to put figures to be compared in a single column rather than in a single row.
3 Where possible use a systematic ordering, for example, by size, so that patterns are easier to spot.
4 Row or column totals and averages will often help interpretation.
5 Row or column percentages will often help comparison, but do make the table more cumbersome.
6 All percentages need either a numerator or denominator; if "75% of patients were cured" there may only have been four patients.
7 In presentation (but not in your original working documents) round figures to two (or exceptionally three) effective digits; later digits are almost always irrelevant and confuse the reader.
8 Include the name and result of any statistical tests you use, preferably without using asterisks, $p < 0.05$, or other statistical jargon.

Example 12—Applying criteria (1)–(4) to table 11.1 would give table 11.2. Applying criteria (5)–(8) to table 11.2 would give table 11.3.

Note that the percentages were calculated from the original figures of table 11.2, not the rounded figures of table 11.3. Also the percentages in the bottom row of table 11.3 add up to 99% because they have been rounded to the nearest whole number. Similarly the rounded figures within table 11.3 do not add up

Table 11.2—Patient numbers by doctor and age group 1994

Doctor	Age group			Total
	64 or less	65–74	75 or more	
PJD	1597	180	132	1909
DAH	1274	213	205	1692
MAP	991	178	154	1323
AGD	564	54	28	646
Total	4426	625	519	5570

Table 11.3—Patient numbers by doctor and age group 1994

Doctor	Age group						Total
	64 or less		65–74		75 or more		
	No	%	No	%	No	%	
PJD	1600	84	180	9	130	7	1900
DAH	1300	75	210	13	200	12	1700
MAP	990	75	180	13	150	12	1300
AGD	560	87	54	8	28	4	650
Total	4400	79	620	11	520	9	5600

Differences between doctors are significant at the 0·1% level (chi-squared = 86 with six degrees of freedom).

exactly to the row and column totals. Including percentages in table 11.3 has highlighted the differences between the age distributions of patients registered with the four doctors. The result of the significance test has confirmed the visual impression that the four distributions differ considerably.

The case for and against graphs

As an alternative, the numbers in a table may be presented graphically. Graphs are useful in highlighting one or two features. They are particularly good at illustrating trends. As a graph cannot include as much detail as a table without becoming confusing, however, you will have to select the information to be presented.

The main disadvantage of graphs is, however, their ability to mislead. Although badly presented tables are difficult to interpret, badly presented graphs are easy to misinterpret. Examples of pitfalls are given on pages 52–57 of Hill and Hill,[6] originally written some time ago but unfortunately still relevant.

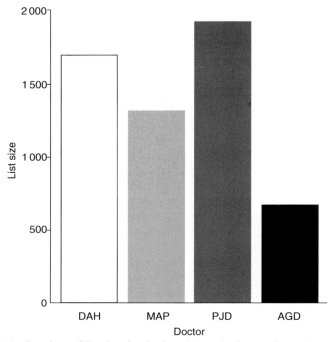

Fig 11.1—Bar chart of list sizes for the four doctors in the practice, 1994

How to present graphs

1 Decide what features of the data you want to highlight; it is better to use two graphs each with a clear message than to combine them in one overcrowded picture.

2 Give the graph a title that is clear and concise.

3 Choose an appropriate type of graph for the data you want to present:

    (a)   the most versatile method is the *bar chart*; fig 11.1 shows a simple bar chart of the list sizes for the four doctors in table 11.1;

    (b)   for variety in presenting categorical data (where patients are classified rather than measured), you may prefer a *pie chart*; fig 11.2 shows the same information as fig 11.1;

    (c)   a *line graph* is the other common alternative to the bar chart;

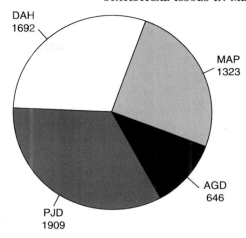

DAH
1692

MAP
1323

AGD
646

PJD
1909

Fig 11.2—Pie chart of list sizes for the four doctors in the practice, 1994

this should not be used for categorical data (for example, list sizes) but only for measured data, where the horizontal scale represents ordered measurements, for example, age or year.

All three types of graph can, with appropriate software, be prepared on a personal computer.

4 Choose between numbers and percentages. This depends on the feature to be highlighted; for the data of table 11.3, for example, do you want to emphasise total workload (numbers) or case mix (percentages)? Percentages provide the better comparison between the practices of different doctors or partnerships. Fig 11.3 is a bar chart with four doctor specific bars for each age group, where the height of each bar represents the percentage of each doctor's patients who belong to that age group. Note that, although complex, this graph does not include the relative sizes of the four doctors' lists.

5 To highlight time trends use a line graph rather than a bar chart. Time trends are well suited to graphical methods; the corresponding tables are harder to read and make it more difficult to identify the main features of the data. Fig 11.4 shows results from table 13.6 (page 210) in graphical form. Differences in trends between three different financial indices are clearly seen, in part because two other indices have been excluded.

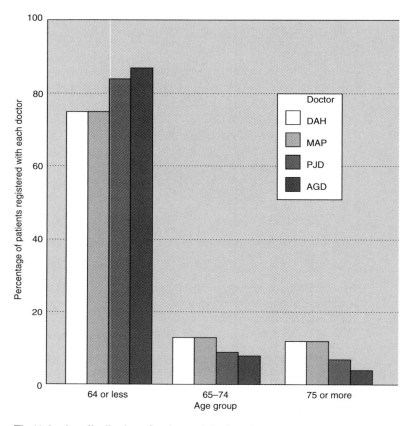

Fig 11.3—Age distribution of patients of the four doctors, 1994

6 Add only enough labels to convey all essential information; in particular label both horizontal and vertical axes, and provide a scale for each.

Conclusion

Our coauthors have argued that medical audit has great potential to improve primary medical care in the United Kingdom. We believe that both its validity and its effectiveness can be enhanced by careful attention to the basic statistical principles of sampling, data validation, analysis, and presentation.

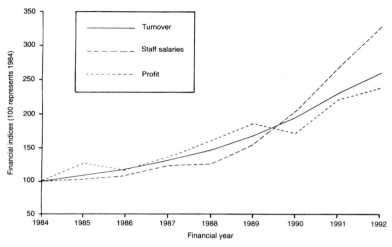

Fig 11.4—Financial trends in the practice, 1984–92

1 Moser CA, Kalton G. *Survey methods in social investigation*, 2nd edn. Aldershot: Gower, 1971.
2 Bland M. *An introduction to medical statistics*. Oxford: Oxford University Press, 1987.
3 Jamieson MJ, Webster J, Phillips S, *et al*. Measurement of blood pressure: Sitting or supine? Once or twice? *J Hypertension* 1990;**8**:635–40.
4 Speight ANP, Lee DA, Hay EN. Underdiagnosis and undertreatment of asthma in childhood. *BMJ* 1983;**286**:1256–8.
5 Gardner MJ, Altman DG. *Statistics with confidence*. London: British Medical Journal, 1989.
6 Hill AB, Hill ID. *Bradford Hill's principles of medical statistics*, 12th edn. London: Edward Arnold, 1991.

Appendix: Calculations for the statistical tests and confidence intervals on pages 174–176

Background to Example 10

The practice standard for the proportion of adult male patients who have had their blood pressure recorded within the past five years has been set at 70%. In one random sample A of 100 such patients, 60 records show such a reading; in another random sample B of 40 such patients, 24 records show such a reading.

Theory

The theory for this example is based on the normal approximation to the binomial distribution (Chapter 7 of Bland[2]).

Assume that a random sample of size n from a population, in which the overall proportion of successes is π, contains r successes. Then the *sample proportion* ($p = r/n$) will have an average of π, although in an individual sample it may be larger or smaller. The larger the sample size, the closer to π the sample proportion is likely to be. The variability of the sample proportion is measured by its standard error—a measure of the likely difference between sample and population proportions. The formula for this standard error is:

$$\sqrt{[\pi(1 - \pi)/n]}.$$

Statistical tests for Example 10

In sample A, $n = 100$, $r = 60$, $\pi = 0.7$ (70%) and $p = 60/100 = 0.6$ (60%). Hence the standard error of the sample proportion is

$$\sqrt{(0.7 \times 0.3/100)} = \sqrt{0.0021} = 0.046 \ (4.6\%).$$

The actual sample proportion of 0·6 (60%) is 0·1 (10%) below the agreed standard. To find out how likely such a difference is, we compare the observed difference of 0·1 with the standard error of 0·046 and conclude that the sample proportion is 2·17 standard errors smaller than the population proportion of 0·7 required to meet the standard. A statistical table of the normal distribution (for example, that on page 121 of Bland[2]) shows that a value of 2·17 or higher has a probability of only 0·015 (1·5%). So a sample proportion as low as 60% is unlikely to occur in a sample of 100 patients from a population with an overall success rate of 70%.

In sample B, $n = 40$ and $r = 24$; thus although π is still 70% and p is still 60% ($24/40 = 0.6$), the standard error is larger:

$$\sqrt{(0.7 \times 0.3/40)} = 0.072 \ (7.2\%).$$

Thus the sample proportion is now only 1·39 standard errors smaller than the agreed standard of 0·7. The same statistical table[2] shows that a value of 1·39 or higher has a probability of 0·082 (8·2%).

184

Confidence intervals for Example 10

The upper and lower limits of the confidence intervals given on page 176 can be calculated from an approximate version of the formula above for the standard error, with p (the sample proportion) replacing π. It is 95% certain that the population proportion lies between

$$p - 1\cdot96\ \sqrt{[p(1-p)/n)}\quad\text{and}\quad p + 1\cdot96\ \sqrt{[p(1-p)/n]}.$$

It is 99% certain that the population proportion lies between

$$p - 2\cdot58\ \sqrt{[p(1-p)/n]}\quad\text{and}\quad p + 2\cdot58\ \sqrt{[p(1-p)/n]}.$$

Confidence levels other than 95% or 99% can be obtained by replacing the multipliers $1\cdot96$ and $2\cdot58$ by another from the same statistical table.[2]

For sample A:

$$p = 0\cdot6\quad\text{and}\quad \sqrt{[p(1-p)/n]} = \sqrt{[0\cdot6 \times 0\cdot4/100]} = 0\cdot049$$

giving 95% confidence limits of $(0\cdot6 - 1\cdot96 \times 0\cdot049)$ and $(0\cdot6 + 1\cdot96 \times 0\cdot049)$, that is, $0\cdot504$ (50·4%) and $0\cdot696$ (69·6%); and the 99% limits are $(0\cdot6 - 2\cdot58 \times 0\cdot049)$ and $(0\cdot6 + 2\cdot58 \times 0\cdot049)$, that is, $0\cdot475$ and $0\cdot725$.

Similarly, for sample B:

$$p = 0\cdot6\quad\text{and}\quad \sqrt{[p(1-p)/n]} = \sqrt{[0\cdot6 \times 0\cdot4/40]} = 0\cdot077$$

giving 95% confidence limits of $0\cdot449$ and $0\cdot751$, and 99% confidence limits of $0\cdot400$ and $0\cdot800$. These limits are wider than those for sample A because of the smaller sample size.

12 Small group work

MARSHALL MARINKER, MAIRI SCOTT

What is a small group? Definitions abound and contradict one another but for the purposes of this chapter we shall define it as a group of between five and 15 people who meet to carry out some agreed enterprise. Eight is often considered the optimum number. These figures are not as arbitrary as might be thought. If the group becomes too small—four or fewer—the possibility of different interactions limits creativity, encourages the taking of fixed roles, and creates too cramped a space for strong feelings to be safely aired or for strong personalities to be moderated by group behaviour. Too large a number and the cohesion of the group begins to break up; for example, it becomes impossible for all the members of a large group to be aware of the behaviour of all the others. In particular, whoever leads a small group must be aware of the behaviour of all of its members. If he or she cannot remain in visual contact with all the members, is unable to notice the eagerness of one, the melancholy of another, the puzzlement or anger or frustration that any group member may exhibit at any time, it will be impossible to address the given task or to deal with the problems within the group that this task may engender.

In the one to one relationship between mother and child, husband and wife, and master and apprentice there can be a passion, a connectedness, an acuteness of feeling that cannot be replicated with the same intensity beyond the private confines of a two person "group." Small groups can certainly generate their own emotional storms: social psychologists of a variety of schools have suggested how and why these come about and these issues will be raised later in this chapter. But there is also something about the configuration of a small group that can exercise a profoundly civilising influence on the relationships of its members.

Thinking and feeling

As members of small groups what is required of each of us is that we find a place, a voice, a part to play in a shared enterprise. To achieve this we have to explore the minds, the thinking, and the feeling of a number of other people. If the enterprise of the group is to succeed we have to understand the strengths of others so that we can make these part of our own strength. We have to explore weaknesses but only so that we can compensate for them. None of this is possible unless each individual begins to reflect on the self. What do I know and how do I know it? What are my capacities and what are their limits? What are the values that drive me, the fears that haunt me? Who am I?

For the most part we are born into small groups. As children we are given the opportunity to play in small groups and, although most of our schools force us into the larger crowd of the classroom, schoolchildren play in small groups and team sports echo this primal expression of the hunter band.

In general practice, as in so many other walks of life, small groups abound: partnerships; primary health care teams; the families of patients; professional committees; and of course small group learning in vocational training and continuing medical education. Each of these groups differs from every other in terms of its structure, its distribution of authority, its explicit intentions, and its implicit rules of engagement. And yet each bears a strong family resemblance to all the others.

Small group work depends above all on a sensitivity to personal boundaries. It demands the ability to fit into the organisation and to make appropriate space for others. Each member of the group needs the tolerance of others if he or she is to venture his or her own ideas, ideals, or feelings. Members of the group can best achieve this tolerance by working hard to create tolerance for the ideas, ideals, and feelings of the others.

It should not surprise us that groups so often fail—for example, general practice partnerships can become frozen in glacial antagonisms. Past quarrels and unresolved misunderstandings from years—sometimes from decades—past survive frozen fresh but dead in ice packed hatred. Marriages and families can be like this;

187

so can our medicopolitical committees. Other groups in trouble suggest a different metaphor. Groups can seem stuck in the groove of a cracked record. Some of the members seem mesmerised by the sound of the voices of the others; some are no longer listening; some find good reason to forget the next meeting; too late, someone suggests trying a new record or switching off the machine.

Tasks

In an essay on medical audit one of us (Marinker, 1986)[1] stated that the following functions would be required from those taking part in the process:

- Determining what aspects of current work are to be observed and measured
- Measuring present performance and trends
- Determining priorities in terms of what is to be changed
- Negotiating these priorities with colleagues, including colleagues in other health care professions, and with client groups
- Developing specific standards of care; this will include an evaluation of the results of good empirical research and the logic of argument where objective evidence for choices is scant
- Negotiating these standards with colleagues
- Monitoring and controlling these standards
- Deciding the frequency of reviews
- Deciding the range, category, and number of standards to be subjected to medical audit
- Deciding about intraprofessional, interprofessional, and public accountability
- Exploring the value system that underpins these choices; these values will touch on public and private morality, the personal and public cost of health care, specific cost effectiveness, quality of life, and so on
- Resolving the many conflicts that arise from the expected variety of values expressed and beliefs held.

Many of these functions, particularly those involving cooperative tasks such as negotiating and resolving conflicts, are best tackled in small groups. In general practice we rarely think of the partnership, or even the primary health care team, as a small group. The term "small group" is more usually reserved for more formal occasions, usually concerned with some educational enterprise.

Medical audit, however, is at one and the same time an indispensable management tool for modern general practice, a research into the functioning of the practice, and an intensive learning experience for all who become involved. If medical audit is to become an integral part of clinical practice and practice management, indeed if it is to function as both the intellectual and organisational framework of the practice, those who take part in it will need from time to time to constitute themselves into formal small groups. There is no other way in which the partnership, or the partners together with the practice manager and other key personnel, can discuss their aims for the practice, the priorities that they wish to choose, the aspects of the practice that are to be observed, and so on. Only by developing the skills of small group membership and leadership can the members of the practice become at once efficient, effective, open, and creative.

Work and avoidance

When a group works successfully at its task, when it shares and addresses its avowed aims, there will be few problems about behaviour or group processes. But sometimes, and not infrequently, the dynamics of the group far from helping actually impede good work. What is going on when things go wrong? What should the leader do?

When things go wrong inside a group it is most comfortable to look first for reasons outside. External ascription of such things as fault, blame, or incompetence does more than defend the *amour propre* of members of the group: it allows them to avoid looking at relationships and it may give them an important sense of cohesiveness, which like all seductions may prove misleading.

One influential model of small group dynamics comes from psychoanalysis. Bion[2] talks about *the work group* and *the basic assumption group*. The characteristics of both these groups, he maintains, are usually present at the same time.

The work group is concerned with the avowed aims. Small group learning in psychoanalysis and related psychologies is concerned with what in general practice we would call case discussion. A work group simply discusses the case and its implications. In particular the work group does not change the subject. When the group begins to change the subject Bion describes it as a basic assumption group. The basic assumption group is concerned with

189

a different belief about what it is that the group has come together to do.

Bion identifies three sorts of behaviour in basic assumption groups. The first is *dependency*. Here the group assumes that the leader will be powerful and omniscient. The leader is seen to be there to solve problems. Balint and others suggest that there is an analogy here with the naive relationship between the general practitioner and the consultant—although this sounds rather old fashioned now. The second is described as *flight–fight*. Here the basic assumption is that the group has enemies without and that the role of the leader is to identify external danger and help the group run away from it. Alternatively he or she may locate the enemy and engage the group in a fight. Group cohesiveness is the aim and paranoia the method. Thirdly, Bion describes *pairing*. The manifestation of this is the development of a dialogue or a series of dialogues within the group. If the leader has been identified the dialogue may occur with the leader. Here the basic assumption of the group is that out of such dialogues (which psychoanalysts of course relate to some sort of sexual union) something good and hoped for and fruitful will be born.

It is worth while remembering that the original model stemmed from the attitudes of psychoanalysis and concerned the function of psychoanalytical therapy groups. This must limit the relevance of the model to our current needs. Pierre Turquet and Robert Gosling,[3] writing about Balint seminars, used the model to explain why groups of hard working and sophisticated doctors who had come together to achieve a specific and important task chose to spend a considerable amount of time and effort on a quite different task: the survival and integrity of the group itself.

Small groups and committees

There is a superficial resemblance between small groups and committees; for example, the size of many committees may be similar to the size that we might expect of a small group. Moreover, it is sometimes easier to understand the behaviour of committees not in terms of their agendas, the power of argument, or the elaborate protocols of committee decision taking but more persuasively in terms of basic assumption groups: dependency, flight–fight, pairing, and so on. Despite these superficial resemblances committees and small groups are quite different kinds of human organisation.

For the most part the members of a committee, however committed to their agenda, come to that agenda with outside affiliations. These affiliations may be stronger and more important than the internal affiliation—that is, the affiliation to the other members of the group and to the agenda. An obvious example would be a liaison committee between two professional organisations. Most committees, however, exhibit this conflict between external and internal affiliation. Members of a committee are often elected to represent a variety of associated constituencies. Each of them may legitimately expect to have his or her own geographical, political, or pressure group interests advanced. This is the essence of committee work. But it is quite different from the essence of small group work.

The way in which a task is presented also differs markedly between committee and small group. The intentions of the small group meeting are most usually stated in broad terms. In medical audit the task might be case discussion or constructing a protocol for the management of patients with psoriasis or deciding what the practice would regard as a reasonable policy on accessibility. The task of the small group may be best seen as the intended destination of a journey. The culture of the group will determine how the journey is to be undertaken: what sort of route will be chosen, what sort of equipment required, who will act as scout, who will be in charge of provisions, who will monitor progress. Small group work does not begin with a route map, with an inventory of the necessary equipment and provisions, still less with marching orders. The creativity of the small group, its ability to solve problems in an unusual way, and, most precious of all, its ability pleasantly to surprise itself are based on the assumption that the journey and how it is to be accomplished can be known only when the group starts to work.

Committees have a different kind of task and a quite different approach. The intentions of a committee must be laid out in fine detail in a written agenda. Those of us who have attended committees where this preliminary work has been neglected know only too well that progress soon becomes impossible. Ideally, committee work is supported by detailed documentation and the members of the committee come armed with argument and counter

191

argument. Only in this way can members of the committee be true to their outward affiliations.

It is possible for the same people to come together at one time as a committee and at another time as a small group. Indeed this may be vital for the proper management and development of general practice. Practice meetings concerned with administration and managerial decisions will certainly need the discipline of a committee meeting. A practice meeting concerned with medical audit may well take as its starting point such a vital question as "What is the practice here to do?" The meeting can succeed in tackling such a question only if it functions not as a committee but as a small group.

Nothing illustrates more clearly the difference between committee work and small group work than the difference between committee chairman and group leader. The chairman begins the meeting not only having achieved considerable control over the agenda but with a formulated view about the decisions that have to be taken. In a sense the chairman begins the meeting with a comprehensive, although still concealed, intention about the minutes that are to be written. The task of the committee members is to challenge these implicit minutes and when possible to change them in the direction that each committee member desires. The major tactic of all members of the committee, including its chairman, is advocacy. However urbane the meeting, however restrained the decorum, there is an inherently adversarial relationship between a committee and its chairman. Far from being a criticism of committees this description reveals its important strengths.

Leaders

The relationship between a group leader and the group contrasts sharply with that between the chairperson and the committee. Far from being adversarial the relationship is intended to be cooperative. The tactic of the leader is to ensure that the group works on its agreed task and that it is made aware when there is deviation from that task. He or she should point out why and how the group has started to escape from what it set out to do and so enable it to return to its purpose. The leader is a resource person for the workings of the small group—not necessarily a resource person for the task being undertaken. That role may fall to another member

192

of the group or indeed to all the members. It is important to bear in mind this distinction between the role of leader and the role of resource. The member of the practice who is most knowledgeable about medical audit may not necessarily be the person best equipped to lead the group.

The question of who is to lead the group is a delicate one. There are perhaps four issues that need to be considered when making a choice.

The first issue concerns *status*. Small group leadership may be charismatic, imposed, democratic, or sapiential. Where leadership is charismatic the leader may have a strong and attractive personality—with ability to disarm and persuade. The strengths and weaknesses of such a basis for leadership are self evident. Such leadership can be powerful, but its intentions can be idiosyncratic and self indulgent.

Leadership can be imposed: the leader may be appointed, for example, by a government or a university department. Again there are strengths and weaknesses. In such a situation the leader has clear accountability to the organisation under whose aegis the group is meeting, but because the leadership is imposed it exhibits a rigid fragility.

The leadership may be democratic: the members of the group themselves may choose their leader. There is strength here in the sense of ownership that the group has of its leader—the sense of participation and negotiation. The weakness is that such leadership, if it is perceived to confront or to challenge the group, can be terminated at the will of the group; so the leader is captive to the group's approval.

Leadership can be sapiential: the leader is recognised because he or she has knowledge or skills that the group wishes to acquire. Again the strength is one of ownership, participation, and negotiation. The weakness is that the group members may settle for a teacher–pupil relationship, a dependence from which too much is hoped for, and from which too much disappointment may ensue.

The status of the leader, of course, is never so categorically defined as these four archetypes suggest. The archetypes need constantly to be borne in mind, however, when problems with the leader arise.

The second issue concerns the *performance* of the leader. There are various styles of leadership, and these can profoundly affect

193

both the feelings in the group and the group's ability to solve problems. The leader may exhibit an authoritarian, a sensitive, a forceful, or a *laissez faire* style. There is no such thing as the most effective style. Each group must discover what kind of leadership suits it best. This is quite different from suggesting that each group must discover what kind of leadership is least confronting or most comfortable. Once the leader begins to collude with the group, work is avoided and tensions will rise.

The third issue concerns the *orientation* of the leader. The leader may reveal an orientation towards an individual member of the group or to some particular members; there may be an orientation to the group as a whole and its interactions or there may be an orientation first and foremost to the task that the group has agreed to undertake.

The fourth issue certainly reflects on the personality of the group leader, but it also reflects on the relationship between the leader and the group. What is the *culture* of the group? What are the values, perhaps never stated explicitly or examined critically, that the group expresses?

Groups sometimes exhibit a strong work ethic with the members showing impatience or even intolerance to those who wish to deflect attention from the task in hand. Other groups value relationships far more than the tasks. If a member is in difficulty all attention to the task must stop while a rescue mission is organised, executed, and brought to a successful conclusion.

These descriptions and differences are of course exaggerations, but they may provide some references for the exploration of your own small group work.

Conclusion

This chapter is intended to give only a partial description of small group work and to relate this to the tasks of medical audit. Much of the book is concerned with the ideas of medical audit, the frames of reference that may be used, the intellectual disciplines that have to be exercised. The reader will, however, have already detected behind these explorations of theory the passionate feelings and the strained relationships that are likely to be encountered. Even at the outset, when the partnership begins to think about its priorities, about what is to be audited, about what constitutes good general practice, the deeply held values of each individual must be challenged. What begins as a search for good standards of care for patients may quickly be transformed into a battle of wills between powerful antagonists.

Most groups concerned with medical audit will not be strangers to one another. This is both good and bad news. The good news is that little time needs to be spent on the preliminaries of small group induction: negotiating relationships, presenting abbreviated and acceptable biographies, and marking out territory. The bad news is that all the past feelings of the members about one another, old scores unsettled, hopes disappointed, opposing moral judgments, and so on may come to the surface with renewed force. Not only will there be interpersonal problems of this nature but also problems among members of allied professions. All the vexing questions about gender, status, values, and accountability that characterise the experience of the so called primary health care team will be sharpened by the attempt to carry out medical audit.

If the group is to be successful in medical audit, or for that matter in any other part of the practice's endeavours, it will be helpful to understand what is going on beneath the surface of the discussion. In all this the task of the group leader is remarkably simple and its execution remarkably complex. The task is constantly to remind the members of the group that they are meeting to enhance the quality of the care of patients. What is complex is the means of achieving this without serious damage to the self image and dignity of every member of the group.

There is a limit to what can be learnt about small group work from written theory. As with learning to play a musical instrument or a good game of tennis one learns most by reflection in action. A good group leader can facilitate this reflection but all the members of the group have a part to play. Finally, it is worth remembering that most general practitioners have considerable interpersonal skills, which they deploy in their consultations. For some mysterious reason these skills desert them at meetings with partners or with other members of the primary health care team. Perhaps what we betray in this strange split between our work with patients and our work with colleagues is a naive belief that, although our patients are vulnerable and require understanding, we and our colleagues are tough and strong and must be feared rather than helped. The reader may regard this as a simplistic exaggeration. But if the idea has a ring of truth then it may point the way to a much gentler, much more humane, and in the end far more effective form of small group work within practices. There is no other way to assure the future success of medical audit.

1 Marinker M. Performance review and professional values. In: Pendleton D, Schofield T, Marinker M, eds, *In pursuit of quality.* London: The Royal College of General Practitioners, 1986.
2 Bion WR. *Experience in groups.* London: Tavistock, 1986.
3 Gosling R, Miller DH, Woodhouse D, Turquet PM. *The use of small groups in training.* London: Codicote Press, 1964.

13 Practice reports

MIKE PRINGLE

Introduction

Practice reports are now an established part of the culture of primary care.[1-3] From the first recorded example in Ballymoney Health Centre in 1969 they have developed from a minority pursuit to a feature of most progressive practices today.

Practice reports evolve.[2-4] A practice may start with a short account of its history, its current staff, and a few statistics, often supplied by the Family Health Services Authority (FHSA) or the Prescription Pricing Authority (PPA). Such early reports are quickly produced, and help to provide motivation and reward for effort. The result may lead to both satisfaction at a milestone achieved and dissatisfaction at the many unanswered questions raised.

At the next stage the report may contain prevention and screening rates, consultation rates, and referrals, all of which require data collection, often over a period of one year. Later come accounts of investigation rates, chronic disease audits, and the practice finances. This evolution mirrors the developing information systems and appreciation of the value of information with the practice.

Practice reports vary widely. There may be common elements, but each report will be a disparate product of varying circumstances. As the motivation comes from within the practice and the report is designed primarily to respond to a practice's needs, the contents and presentation can be idiosyncratic. As a practice looks beyond its boundaries it may need to compare itself with other practices and with local and national norms.

To do this there must be common definitions for the items the practice wishes to compare.[3] Although the range and depth of a practice report will be determined by the needs and skills of the practice, there will be an increasing recognition of the value of standardisation for certain aspects.[3]

Even if it fulfils no other role, a practice report must be of value to the practice for the following: measuring the quantity and quality of care;[5] determining the use of, and need for, resources; and setting targets to which the practice can aspire.[6] To do this it must be honest, and honesty creates vulnerability. Each practice must decide how far it is willing to disseminate its report and whether it requires two versions. To be of value, as well as being honest a report must be accurate, which requires the contents to be both quantitative (with numbers, percentages, and averages) and qualitative (with descriptions of how the practice is seen by its members). In addition, it needs to be of sufficient depth to allow a reasoned analysis of the practice's care, its problems, and their solutions.

Over the years practice reports can be used to monitor developments, to record performance against targets, and to identify trends. Just as the computer has become an essential tool for data processing so the annual report is becoming a prerequisite for data presentation and understanding, and thus an integral part of the management of a modern practice.

What is a practice report?

Any document produced by a practice which describes the working of the practice can be described as a practice report. Practice reports have, however, acquired some characteristics.

They are usually produced annually, express a consensus view of the practice team, and are, at the least, available to every member of the team. Their contents may include a description of practice philosophy, the health needs of the patient, an analysis of the practice's delivery of care, an audit of clinical standards, and the setting of targets for the future.

A major confusion has been created by the use of the term "annual report" by the Department of Health in the new contract for general practitioners.[7] Although annual reports can be seen as one specialised form of practice report with overlapping contents, they are clearly philosophically different documents.

Reports to the Family Health Services Committee

Annual reports are now a contractual requirement,[8] so the need is not initiated by the practice and the practice may comply without realising that the information involved will relate to any of its problems. This means that the first prerequisite of the educational audit process, an acknowledgment of a potential problem, is not present. The motivation within a practice for producing the report is contractual compliance, not honest self evaluation.

Contractural annual reports are intended to act as tools for minimum standard monitoring and as a weapon in the cost containment war, which is characterised by government sources as "value for money." Practitioners may unfortunately become wary of presenting information in a straightforward way, not only in annual reports but in any practice reports, because they fear that the information may be used for punitive purposes against either themselves or other practitioners.

Fundholding practices are also required to file regular data reports on the process of care within the practice—especially those involving secondary care services. To any practices these are bureaucratic necessities, but these data can be presented and interpreted meaningfully in a practice report.

Compiling practice reports

In the remainder of this chapter we shall consider practice reports that are compiled voluntarily as an educational, clinical, and management audit. They are intended to throw light on the performance of the practice, both subjectively and objectively, so that the practice may evaluate itself in a spirit of self criticism. Such honesty inevitably creates vulnerability, and the practice will only be prepared to tolerate such vulnerability if the risks are minimised. If there are strong fears that data gathered for internal educational audit could be used for making punitive external judgments—for monitoring the contract, determining earnings, or instituting litigation—practices will have a powerful motive for not preparing practice reports.

A practice needs to be clear about its motivation in writing a report. The main reasons for a report are the following:

- To review the "state of the practice:" the health and needs of the practice population; the quality of health care; and the personnel, the organisation, and the finances of the practice

199

- To review the activities and developments of the past year, including the achievement of previous targets
- To express intentions, both qualitative and numerical, as in targets for the next year
- To act as a tool for business and health care planning
- To boost team morale and aid team building
- To communicate all this to staff, patients, and health authorities
- To act as a historical record of the practice.

Not all these reasons will appeal to every practice but there is no practice that cannot benefit from an examination of its health needs and its provision of care.

The content and format of practice reports are flexible. Practices need to choose where to start and the pace of their progress, but three theoretical stages can be postulated.

Stage 1: description—The practice describes its structure (personnel, premises, patients) and its process (reports from the primary health care team).

Stage 2: process audit—As well as describing itself, the practice audits and publishes its workload—that is, consultations, visits, clinics—referral and investigation rates, prevention levels, and prescribing.

Stage 3: clinical audit—At this level the practice also publishes audits of its clinical protocols for common chronic diseases and special groups of patients.

Although some of the information in the annual report may reappear in the practice report—for example, referral and investigation rates—it will be serving a different purpose in a different context. Here I shall concentrate on the nature of this purpose and attempt to define the context.

What function does a practice report perform?

Internal functions

The prime functions of a practice report should be internal to the practice. If it is compiled with a self conscious look over the shoulder at the possible reactions outside the practice, then its value inside the practice may well be compromised.

The practice report is above all a tool in the management of change. It is a means of addressing the following key questions:[3-5]

- Where have we come from?
- Where are we now?
- Where are we going?
- How do we intend to get there?

Knowing where the practice has been helps in interpreting the present and highlighting trends that may continue. Target setting has to be based on an understanding of the past and the present; deciding how the targets are to be achieved is of course essential.

Some practices go through this process in a somewhat disorganised way without the imposed structure of an annual report. They risk seeing areas of practice activity in a piecemeal fashion and often fail to share their ideas with employees. Worst of all, they risk missing a stage, basing their perception of problems on insufficient data, and applying inappropriate solutions.

For many practices change is not something that they bring about but something that happens to them. They are reactive in a proactive world and this passivity results in their being left increasingly behind. Starting a practice report is one way of changing the culture of a practice from being reactive to proactive.

A practice report has other internal functions. It can inform the staff and patients of the activities of the practice, and it can mark the practice's achievements—it can acknowledge effort and excellence. By increasing awareness and understanding of the practice's goals it can draw the partners, staff, and patients into an involvement that leads to high staff morale, thriving patient groups, a coherent working relationship among partners, and the achievement of targets.

External functions

In setting targets a practice has to make judgments based on the present. Reasoned judgments can be made only if it has access to normative data from other practices with which it can compare its performance. By publishing its report externally each practice will help others to set their norms.

By making practice reports common currency we shall be able to make our peer reviews meaningful. To judge a practice using

201

statements made authoritatively by a central body is a limited exercise, but to compare practices by using the norms of other similar practices gives peer review credibility. It is far better that central norms[9]—for example, as outlined in the Royal College of General Practitioners' guide to assessment for fellowship[10]—should be based on the real performances of real practices.[11]

The need for accountability to our patients[12] is another important motive for preparing practice reports. Although our peers may judge us by the profession's criteria, our patients should be able to judge us by their own criteria. An openness about our performance, whatever the shortcomings of that performance may be, is far better than a smug silence.

Sharing information about our performance with patients creates an awareness in the practice population of its needs. This was precisely the purpose of the Medical Officer of Health's annual report before 1972—an examination of the needs of a population and the extent to which they were met.[13] This public health function is within the grasp of general practices using information technology to generate high quality audits.

The last external function that practice reports can perform is to defend the profession. We are open to the charges that we are not evolving, that we do not set standards, that we are not self critical, that we do not perform, and that we do not communicate with our patients. Practice reports can answer these criticisms both in individual practices and, collectively, at the national level. We have hidden our lights for too long; practice reports are one way of raising the torch.

The areas to be covered in a practice report

Two reports or one?

If a practice report is to stimulate higher standards and a more focused management of change then it must be honest. If such honesty would compromise the practice then the dissemination of the report must be restrained. This might be the case with details of partnership earnings, for example, but could also include any information with direct bearing on compliance with the general practice contract. Every practice should therefore produce an unexpurgated core report. If it decides that this report should not be circulated widely it can either produce a second, limited edition for wider distribution or restrict the single report to a limited readership.

These issues need to be decided before the report is written. If, as happens in my practice, only one version of the report is written and it is available to everyone within the practice, including the patients who read copies put in the waiting room, and outside bodies, including other practices and the FHSA, the style must be suitable for the potential readership. If patients are to read it some terms need defining, and the text needs to be accessible.

Contents

In constructing reports, practices usually start with a few items and build up. The four stages have already been listed. The complexity of the first report and the speed with which it is produced will depend on both the will of the practice and the sophistication of its information systems. The possible contents (table 13.1) are those that a practice might aspire to, and could achieve, at the time.[4]

The examples quoted in the text and the tables are from the seventh practice report (covering April 1993 to March 1994 and published in July 1994) from my own practice in Collingham, Newark, Nottinghamshire. This report is far from perfect and is held up not as a model of perfection but as an example.

Although some items in table 13.1 are self explanatory, others need elaboration. The practice should set out the philosophy, services, and key aspirations in *the practice objectives* section. It is against these that the report as a whole will be judged.

We like to present the numerical material in graphic form when appropriate, as shown in figs 13.1–13.3. Causes of death can be interesting (table 13.2) to patients and doctors alike, and the number of patients with selected major diagnoses are important in assessing need and planning care (table 13.3), as well as just patient numbers (table 13.4).

Lifestyle data can be presented in tabular form (table 13.5) or graphically as in fig 13.4.

In the quality of care section we present our charter standards and their audit, and report on our quality assurance programme. This includes auditing of significant events (see box on page 208).

Every partner eagerly awaits the analysis of workload (figs 13.5 and 13.6) if only to check on equity (fig 13.7).

Table 13.1—The contents of a practice report

Introduction

The practice's objectives
—its mission statement and role

The health needs of our patients
—population profile (age, sex, location, etc)
—population changes (deaths, births, turnover)
—prevalence of major diagnoses
—lifestyle information
—socioeconomic data (from the census)
—special health needs of the practice population

The quality of care delivered to our patients
—results of clinical and managerial audits
—the practice's policies for delivery of care and its range of services
—the practice's patients' charter standards and their audit
—the practice's future plans for enhancing quality of care

Our delivery of care
—members of staff
—reports from team members
—workload (consultation rates, referrals, investigations, and preventive activity)
—financial report
—the future *plans for the delivery of care*

A review of the year
—main events of the year
—meetings
—education and training

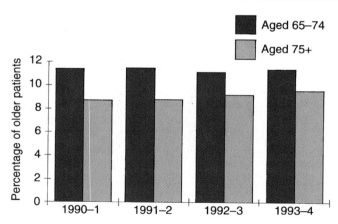

Fig 13.1—The proportion of patients aged 75 years and over is increasing

A vital part of any practice report should be *reports from members of the primary health care team*—the doctors, receptionists, practice

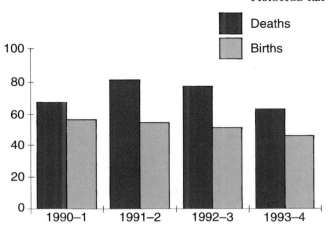

Fig 13.2—The local birth rate is slowly falling. The fertility rate (number of births per 1000 women aged 15–44) is also declining from a high of 62·1 in 1991–2 to 47·5 in 1993–4. This shows that the falling birth rate is not the result of fewer eligible women, but less fertility. There are consistently more deaths than births

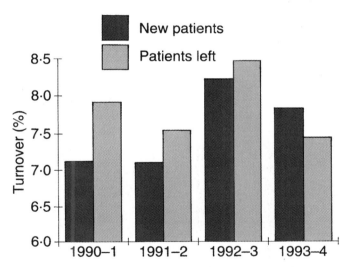

Fig 13.3—Although there is a tendency for the turnover to increase in recent years, the Collingham practice is still a lower turnover practice compared with many

and district nurses, health visitors, the school nurse, the counsellor, and in our case the attached physiotherapist. These reports can be linked to the report from the patient participation group to give a

205

Table 13.2—Causes of death*

Cause of death	1990–1	1991–2	1992–3	1993–4
Cancer	21	15	20	16
Stroke	6	27	8	6
Respiratory disease	14	20	10	10
Heart disease	17	3	22	16
Old age	3	8	4	5
Other	5	8	13	9
Total	66	81	77	62

* These show no coherent pattern (and there is doubt about the accuracy of the 1991–2 allocation between stroke and heart disease).

Table 13.3—A look at some major diagnoses in the practice*

Major diagnoses	Number of patients
Diabetes mellitus	105
Asthma	
Total	377
Number on treatment in past two years	246
Hypertension (high blood pressure)	334
Ischaemic heart disease (angina, heart attack, etc)	226
Osteoarthritis of knees	113
Dementia	23
Glaucoma	34
Depression (ever recorded)	196
Multiple sclerosis	17
Stroke	
Ever	74
In past two years	20

* This shows that 1·9% of the practice population has diabetes, 6·8% asthma, 6·0% hypertension, 4·1% ischaemic heart disease, and 3·5% have been recorded as suffering from depression.

Table 13.4—Patient numbers

Doctor	Patients' age (1994) years			Totals	
	<65	65–74	75 +	1993	1994
DAH	1274	213	205	1682	1692
MAP	991	178	154	1381	1323
PJD	1597	180	132	1848	1909
AGD	564	54	28	661	646
Totals	4426	625	519	5572	5570

206

Table 13.5—Smoking data of practice, and the national target

	Collingham	National target by year 2000
Percentage adults with smoking status recorded (aged 16 and over)	84·5	
Percentage current smokers (aged 16 and over)	21·7	20
Percentage pregnant women with smoking status recorded	100	
Percentage pregnant women current smokers	23	A third stopping at start of pregnancy
Percentage teenagers with smoking recorded	3·7	
Percentage teenagers smoking	0·2	6

We have much less smoking among adults than the national average (28% of females; 31% of males), but we have not started recording teenager smoking or alcohol consumption. The national targets are those set by the Department of Health in "The Health of the Nation."

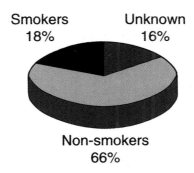

Smokers
18%

Unknown
16%

Non-smokers
66%

Fig 13.4—The smoking status of adults expressed graphically

descriptive picture of the workings of the practice from both sides of the reception desk.

The extent to which a practice wants to include *financial data* in its report will vary. If a separate report is being prepared for the partners only then can it include the full financial details, but as these are usually a duplicate of the accountant's report this may be unnecessary. It is, however, possible to highlight trends by using an arbitrary year as a base (equal to 100 as in retail price indices) and showing changes year by year as in table 13.6. Data presented in this manner should be publishable to any readership.

The practice reports on its significant event auditing activity

The Collingham practice has demonstrated its commitment to high quality care by having regular significant event audit meetings over the past three years. Each doctor, nurse, and manager records any event that happens which might give insight into the life of the practice. These would include every time one of the following occurs:

- A new diagnosis of cancer
- A new heart attack or stroke
- An urgent visit to a patient with asthma, diabetes, or epilepsy
- An unplanned pregnancy
- A visit requested but not done
- A patient complaint
- A patient leaves the practice without changing address
- A prescribing or dispensing error

Each event is discussed openly in a meeting to which all the doctors, nurses, and managers are invited. The medical notes are examined, the care given is analysed, and the implications for the practice discussed. There are four outcomes from these discussions:

1 *Celebration*	Where, as is often the case, the care given was perfectly satisfactory, then the people involved are congratulated—something that happens all too seldom in busy practices
2 *A conventional audit*	Sometimes we are unsure how to react to an event—we don't know if the problem is common and whether a change in policy would be justified. On these occasions, the practice does a numerical audit and then re-discusses the issue
3 *Immediate action*	In some cases a shortfall in the delivery of care is identified which is sufficiently important and common to justify an immediate agreement to change our behaviour or our systems
4 *No action*	Many of the events discussed are handled adequately and routinely. They do not highlight quality issues and we cannot learn lessons from them

The power of these case based discussions to heighten our awareness of quality issues is often greater than that of conventional audits. The emotional content of the discussions makes behavioural change more likely, and the celebration of success rewards high standards. The perceived value of these meetings was clearly illustrated by the fact that they were recently increased to monthly.

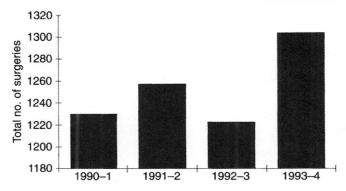

Fig 13.5—There has been a clear increase in the number of surgeries offered this year

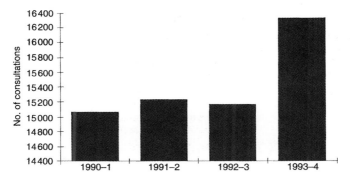

Fig 13.6—The number of consultations with the doctors in the practice has risen in line with the number of surgeries

Creating a practice report

Who does the work?

Creating a practice report may at first seem a daunting task. The work, however, is not onerous when split among many members of the team.

The first report can skimp on statistics and concentrate on description. Each member of the team can be asked to write a report on his or her past year, and figures that are available from the FHSA and the Prescription Pricing Authority can be added. The advantage of this approach is that it allows a short lead in time from decision to product.

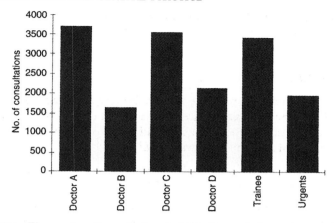

Fig 13.7—The number of consultations in 1993–4 by each doctor. Doctors B and D are job sharers. When surgeries are fully booked, urgent cases are seen at the end by those doctors finishing first. They are therefore not allocated to individual doctors when the totals are generated

Table 13.6—The financial health of the practice presented in a confidential but informative manner

	1984	1985	1986	1987	1988	1989	1990	1991	1992
Turnover	100	108	117	131	147	168	196	232	261
Total expenditure	100	98	118	128	140	148	208	236	267
Staff salaries + pensions	100	102	108	123	125	155	206	269	329
Office expenses (including telephone)	100	111	126	161	166	165	207	219	240
Profit	100	127	116	137	161	187	172	222	240
Profit as percentage of turnover	35	41	34	36	38	38	30	33	33

It is then crucial to decide what information is needed for the next report. Many items can be collected by using simple recording sheets or by multicolour computer entries.

Information systems can involve everybody in the practice, but only a small amount of extra effort is needed from each. The receptionists, for example, can record appointments and visits totals for checking against the computer analyses.

In our practice one partner is editor of the practice report, the practice manager encourages and cajoles the authors of each section, and the data analyst (a full time member of staff) prepares the routine practice statistics. As the data are seen within the practice to be valuable for planning and monitoring, no one resents the time put in and the act of publishing rewards those who have collected the data for their efforts over the year.

Definition of data items

It is important for practices to use the few common definitions in their reports to facilitate interpretation and comparison.[3] To this end, these common definitions should be followed, but a fuller set has been published by Howarth et al.[15]

A fully registered National Health Service patient is someone who is fully registered with the family practitioner committee.

This statement may sound self evident, but practices using computers often include patients on their list as soon as they hand in their cards and exclude them as soon as it is known that they have moved. In a practice with a high turnover but a static total population this should give approximately the same number of patients, but the time lag means that the identity of these patients may vary by up to 10%.

To achieve consistency it is necessary to use the same patient base as the FHSA, and this means that the practice must make retrospective adjustments to the date of registration notified by the committee.

Any grouping of patients by age should specify the date of the grouping (usually the first day of a quarter) and it should include those patients who are of the specified age on the specified date.

If, for example, a practice states in its report that it has 80 children aged five and it used these as the denominator for immunisations, this could have a number of meanings. It could mean the number of children aged five on the first day of the year or at the time of the audit report. It could mean all those children who were aged five at any point in the year or those who had a fifth birthday in the year. To avoid confusion it is therefore necessary to follow the rule set out above.

Any subgroup may be excluded from a grouping provided the criteria for exclusion are explicit and data for the whole group are given.

If a practice wishes to give the immunisation rate for children born into the practice (as distinct from those who move in after birth) it is quite at liberty to do so. It should, however, give the

211

figures for all the children and clearly define the exclusion criterion used in working out the figure for the subgroup.

The date entered for a procedure is the date on which it is carried out; the date of a diagnosis is the date when it was first made, with reasonable certainty.

This rule means that a blood test, for example, is dated from when the sample is taken, not from when the result is received. A diagnosis is dated from the moment that it is made, not from the date when the patient joined the practice with a pre-existing diagnosis, or from the date on which the diagnosis was entered in the problem list or disease register.

Age grouped data should normally be presented in single years, in five year bands, or aggregates of five year bands in the series 0–4, 5–9, 10–14, and so on.

This may be self evident but is easily forgotten when auditing an adult group. There is a strong temptation to lapse into bands of, for example, 36–45.

Computers

Although a practice report can, of course, be produced manually, a computer will ease the burden of work, increase the scope, and improve the accuracy of the data.

Computers are, of course, only as good as the information entered and the program used. Many items—for example, referrals—can be quite easily recorded manually but others—for example, prevention uptake rates—are laborious to calculate manually and can be done rapidly and accurately by a computer.

A computer can also be used as a word processor and to generate graphics to help in the presentation of data.

The future

Practice reports are becoming more sophisticated. The reason for this is that the management of the health service is becoming more complex and the professional requirement for general practitioners to demonstrate quality of care is more pressing.

As a tool for management and quality demonstration the practice report will increasingly be looked upon as an essential part of primary care. Its scope will increase not in response to a desire for self exhibition but as a way to meet the challenges of an evolving health service.

As the complexity of practice reports increases so will their uniformity.[3] This is not to say that they will become drab, repetitive documents, but that they will contain key tables which can be compared with data from previous years and with those from other practices. This will be particularly important when practices work together to commission care, as is already occurring with multifunding. If a practice is to increase its ability to attract resources it will need to cooperate with other practices in the same area. This will mean aggregating data, and some supplementary mutual data gathering—for example, of patient need.

Conclusions

In this chapter I have attempted to define and to justify practice reports. The range of material to be included and how to set about producing a report have been considered. It is of course for each practice to decide how, or whether, to proceed.

If general practitioners are to avoid ever widening state involvement in clinical areas they will need to develop skills in the formulation and presentation of ideas and information One stop, perhaps the major step, along this road is the production of high quality practice reports, and I for one look to the day when they will be part of every practice's activity.

1 Urquhart AS. Practice annual reports. *J R Coll Gen Pract* 1987;**37**: 148.

2 Wilson A, Jones S, O'Dowd TC. Survey of practice annual reports. *J R Coll Gen Pract* 1989;**39**:250–2.

3 Wilton J. A review of general practice reports: the need for standardisation. *BMJ* 1990;**300**:851–3.

4 Gray DJP. Practice annual reports. In: Gray DJP, Gray JP, eds, *The medical annual 1985.* Bristol: Wright, 1985:2282–300.

5 Metcalf DHH. Audit in general practice. *BMJ* 1989;**299**:1293–4.

6 Keeble BR, Chivers CA, Gray JAM. The practice annual report: post mortem or prescription? *J R Coll Gen Pract* 1989;**39**:467–9.

7 Department of Health. *General practice in the National Health Service: the 1990 contract.* London: Department of Health, 1989.

8 Department of Health. *Terms of service for doctors in general practice.* London: Department of Health, 1989.

9 Royal College of General Practitioners. *Report from general practice 23: What sort of doctor?* London: RCGP, 1985.

10 Royal College of General Practitioners. *Guide to assessment for fellowship of the Royal College of General Practitioners.* London: RCGP, 1989.

11 Baker R. *Practice assessment and quality of care.* London: Royal College of General Practitioners, 1989. (Occasional paper 39.)

12 Hart JT. *A new kind of doctor.* London: Merlin Press, 1988:237–41.

13 Black N. Annual reports on public health. *BMJ* 1989;**299**:1059–60.

14 Pritchard P, ed. *Patient participation in general practice.* London: Royal College of General Practitioners, 1981. (Occasional paper 17.)

15 Jarman B. Identification of underprivileged areas. *BMJ* 1983;**286**: 1705–9.

16 Howarth FP, Maitland JM, Duffus PRS. Standardisation of core data for practice annual reports: a pilot study. *J R Coll Gen Pract* 1989;**39**: 463–6.

Further reading

Cembrowicz S. How to write a practice annual report. *BMJ* 1989;**298**: 953–4.

Westcott R, Jones RVH, eds. *Information handling in general practice.* London: Croom Helm, 1988.

Index

215

Also from the BMJ Publishing Group

CONTROVERSIES IN HEALTH CARE POLICIES: CHALLENGES TO PRACTICE
Edited by Marshall Marinker

Controversies in Health Care Policies: Challenges to Practice is the result of the work of six think tanks of clinical experts, GPs, managers, and patient representatives. It documents a unique investigation into the burning controversies in old age and disease; medical practice variation; rational prescribing; primary care following Tomlinson; risk in medicine; and public access to medical information, and comes up with innovative and realistic ideas for the way forward.
ISBN 0 7279 0894 4

OUTCOMES INTO CLINICAL PRACTICE
Edited by Tony Delamothe

Outcomes research, the new buzz word in health care, refers to the generation, collection, and analysis of the results of medical care. Such information offers the opportunities to improve clinical effectiveness and set standards for good practice. Based on a ground breaking conference held by the *BMJ*, BMA, and UK Clearing House, *Outcomes into Clinical Practice* discusses the issues involved and gives real examples of how outcomes research works best.
ISBN 0 7279 0888 X

CHANGE AND TEAMWORK IN PRIMARY CARE
Edited by Mike Pringle

General practice is now at the centre of the health service and this book addresses the vital challenges confronting those working in it. In the first part experts describe with real examples the skills required for managing change and in the second the tasks and relationships within the new primary health care teams are examined.

"In a time of unprecedented and unrelenting change of primary care, this is a very welcome book."
Health Education Journal
ISBN 0 7279 0779 4

QUALITY AND SAFETY IN ANAESTHESIA
Edited by Jonathan Secker Walker

With contributions from leading figures in anaesthetic audit, this concise book addresses the quality and management of risk; critical incidents and human factors in anaesthesia; standards for routine monitoring; standards in training; managing a department; resource management; and computers.
ISBN 0 7279 0828 6

For further details of this book and our full range of titles write to Marketing Department, BMJ Publishing Group, BMA House, Tavistock Square, London WC1H 9JR or telephone 0171 383 6541.